# Case Studies in
# Cardiology
# for the
# House Officer

# Case Studies in Cardiology for the House Officer

Edited by

## Joel W. Heger, M.D.

Getzen, Heger & Conrad Cardiology Group
Pasadena, California

## Neil W. Treister, M.D.

Ukiah, California

## Steven L. Writer, M.D.

Boise, Idaho

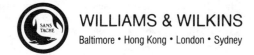

## WILLIAMS & WILKINS

Baltimore • Hong Kong • London • Sydney

*Editor:* Kimberly Kist
*Associate Editor:* Victoria M. Vaughn
*Copy Editor:* Bill Cady
*Design:* Bob Och
*Production:* Raymond E. Reter
*Cover Design:* Dan Pfisterer

Copyright © 1988
Williams & Wilkins
428 East Preston Street
Baltimore, MD 21202, USA

Accurate indications, adverse reactions, and dosage schedules for drugs are provided
in this book, but it is possible that they may change. The reader is urged to review
the package information data of the manufacturers of the medications mentioned.

*Printed in the United States of America*

**Library of Congress Cataloging in Publication Data**

Heger, Joel W.
    Case studies in cardiology for the house officer / Joel W. Heger,
    Neil Treister, Seven L. Writer. p.          cm.          Includes bibliographies and index.
    ISBN 0-683-03945-8
        1. Heart—Diseases—Case studies.   I. Treister, Neil.   II. Writer, Steven L.   III.
Title. [DNLM: 1. Cardiovascular Diseases—diagnosis—case studies. WG141
H462c]        RC682.H39 1988        616.1′2075—dc 19
    DNLM/DLC for Library of Congress                                        88-14306
                                                                                                    CIP

                                                89   90   91   92
                        2   3   4   5   6   7   8   9   10

# Series Editor's Foreword

The series, Case Studies for the House Officer, has been designed to teach medicine by a case study approach. It is considered a supplement to the parent House Officer Series which provides information in a problem-oriented format. Cardiology for the House Officer has proved particularly popular with house officers and medical students. In Case Studies in Cardiology for the House Officer, Drs. Heger, Treistor, and Writer have compiled an impressive series of interesting cases that cover most common cardiac problems. They have added thoughtful "Pearls" and "Pitfalls" and pertinent electrocardiograms and echocardiograms. The book should be a useful and enjoyable learning experience for students of cardiology.

Lawrence P. Levitt, M.D.
Senior Consultant in Neurology
Lehigh Valley Hospital Center
Allentown, Pennsylvania

Clinical Professor of Neurology
Hahnemann University

# *Preface*

This collection of cases is a response to the enthusiastic reception given to Cardiology for the House Officer, which appeared in its first edition in 1982 and second edition in 1987. We have used that book extensively in teaching medical students and house officers and have recognized the need for a problem-oriented case series that would emphasize our approach to the diagnosis and management of patients with cardiac disease. Case Studies in Cardiology for the House Officer is a synthesis of what we have learned from our patients in the practice of cardiology and from our students in clinical training.

Our goal has been to provide an enjoyable and readable text that helps students assess their own level of understanding of many of the important concepts in cardiology. We have included cases from our practices that represent the most commonly encountered problems in ischemic, valvular, myopathic, congenital and other forms of heart disease.

The cases are presented in summary form with concise histories, pertinent physical findings and important laboratory data. The questions are aimed at assessing the house officer's ability to recognize problems and make clinical decisions. The pearls and pitfalls included with each case will supplement the reader's fund of knowledge. The references are carefully chosen to provide in-depth review.

This collection of cases is not intended to provide a comprehensive review of cardiology, nor does it stress controversial issues. Furthermore, when presenting case studies we realize there is a tendency to oversimplify and to avoid extremely complex problems, and we ask for the reader's understanding of these limitations.

# Acknowledgments

The authors wish to thank the patients whose clinical stories are represented in this book.

We are grateful to our families for their understanding, patience and encouragement.

We would also like to thank Laura Treister for her outstanding work in preparation of the manuscript.

# Contents

## CASE 1: NEW ONSET OF CHEST PAIN

HISTORY

A 48-year-old meat packer presents to the emergency room with exertionally induced substernal chest pressure radiating to the jaw and lasting 5 minutes. There is no diaphoresis, dyspnea or nausea. He has no previous history of cardiac problems but has had 4 or 5 such episodes in the past 2 months. He has smoked cigarettes for 20 years and has 2 older brothers with coronary artery disease.

EXAMINATION

The patient's blood pressure is 140/90; his heart rate is 85. The physical examination is otherwise unremarkable, with the exception of bilateral arcus corneae and a 4th heart sound.

ADDITIONAL DATA

The lab work and chest x-ray are normal.

The ECG is shown below:

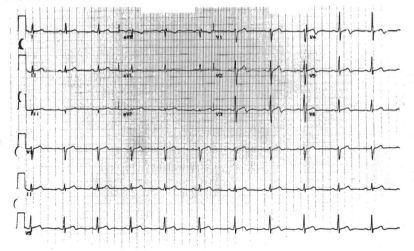

INTERPRETATION OF ECG: Biphasic T waves over the anterior precordium; otherwise normal.

QUESTIONS

1. What is the most likely underlying diagnosis?
2. What coronary artery is most likely involved?
3. What therapy would be most reasonable at this time?
4. If the patient has further symptoms on medical therapy, what other steps should be taken?

ANSWERS

1. Angina pectoris. The important risk factors of a positive family history, smoking, and the absence of physical findings compatible with valvular, congenital or myopathic disease strongly favor coronary artery disease as the underlying etiology.

2. This particular ECG pattern of biphasic T waves over the anterior precordium is very suggestive of a significant stenosis in the left anterior descending coronary artery.

3. Comprehensive medical therapy for angina involves the use of nitrates, beta blockers and calcium channel blockers. Although many patients can get relief with only one or a combination of 2 of these types of agents, some patients seem to require use of all 3 drug types:

   (a) Nitrates were the first class of drugs prescribed for the prevention and treatment of angina. There is a wide variety of nitrate compounds available which can be dispensed orally, sublingually, topically or intravenously. A reasonable, cost-effective approach to start treatment in this patient would be to use isosorbide dinitrate 10-20 mg p.o. q.i.d. Sublingual nitrates may be used before activities that provoke angina.

   (b) Beta blockers (either selective or nonselective) are effective in angina treatment because they decrease the myocardial oxygen demand by lowering the heart rate and blood pressure (double product). Many beta blockers are available. This patient was treated with atenolol 50 mg p.o. q.d., which was attractive to both the patient and his doctor in that it could be given once a day and seemed to have no adverse side effects in this case. Certainly another selective beta blocker, such as metoprolol, or a nonselective agent, such as propranolol or timolol, would be reasonable to use in this patient.

   (c) Calcium channel blockers are the newest addition in the medical therapy for angina. The 3 currently available choices include nifedipine, verapamil and diltiazem. Nifedipine is the most powerful arterial vasodilator and hence would often be the calcium blocker of choice in a hypertensive patient; the average dose is 10 mg p.o. t.i.d. to q.i.d. Verapamil has the greatest effect on AV nodal conduction and would be the drug of choice if the patient has paroxysmal atrial tachycardia; the average dose is 80-120 mg p.o. t.i.d. to q.i.d. Diltiazem is often the best tolerated if there are no reasons to choose one drug over another; the average dose is 30-60 mg p.o. t.i.d. to q.i.d.

4. With continued limiting symptoms on medical therapy, this patient should have coronary angiography to consider other forms of treatment, such as angioplasty (PTCA) or coronary bypass surgery (CABG).

## PEARLS

1. Since angina is a diagnosis made on historical grounds, it is important to establish the characteristics of the chest discomfort--usually described as tightness, pressure or heaviness. Because the word "pain" can be misleading to some patients, we choose to avoid it in many interview situations.
2. Anginal discomfort is usually precipitated by exercise or emotional upset and relieved by rest or nitroglycerin.
3. Medical therapy of angina has improved greatly in the past decade; optimal medical therapy, including nitrates and beta and calcium channel blockers, will result in marked improvement or complete relief of symptoms in many patients.
4. Angioplasty has emerged as a powerful tool in the symptomatic relief of patients with coronary artery disease.
5. Angina accompanied by ECG changes has a worse prognosis than angina with no ECG changes and is predictive of a 20-30% occurrence of a significant cardiac event (myocardial infarction, unstable angina, need for CABG or PTCA) in the ensuing 6 months.

## PITFALLS

1. Patients with classic angina may have normal coronary arteries. This situation may occur when the heart is subjected to acute or chronic increases in workload, such as aortic stenosis, hypertrophic cardiomyopathy or hypertension.
2. There are some patients who have angina, normal coronary arteries, and no abnormalities which increase myocardial workload. The diagnosis for these patients has been called "syndrome X" because of its enigmatic nature.
3. Many patients with angina will have normal ECG's at rest.
4. In a given individual, angina may occur with varying amounts of exercise and at different times of the day. This variable threshold appears to be due to changes in vasomotor tone.

5. The continuous, chronic use of nitrates may result in decreasing effects of the drugs (tolerance).

## REFERENCES

Chatterjee K, Rouleau JL, Parmley WW:  Medical management of patients with angina.  JAMA 252:1170, 1984.

Levine HJ:  Mimics of coronary heart disease.  Postgrad Med 64:58, 1978.

Reeves TJ, Oberman A, Jones WA, et al:  Natural history of angina pectoris. Am J Cardiol 33:423, 1974.

**CASE 2: ACCELERATING EPISODES OF CHEST PAIN**

HISTORY

A 65-year-old engineer presents with a 3-week history of multiple bouts of severe chest pressure. The patient has a history of a myocardial infarction (MI) 5 years ago and has had occasional anginal pains in the past year. Over the week prior to presentation his episodes of chest discomfort have become more severe, more frequent and of longer duration. The patient noted that he was using more nitroglycerin tablets but getting less relief. He has a long history of hypertension. He is an adult-onset diabetic and has been a heavy smoker for many years. There is no history of hypercholesterolemia.

EXAMINATION

Physical examination reveals a well-developed male with a blood pressure of 150/95, a pulse of 85 and respirations of 16. He has a regular rate and rhythm with a prominent S4. No cardiomegaly is noted, and no heart murmur is heard. His lungs are clear to auscultation. There is no peripheral edema.

ADDITIONAL DATA

Laboratory data reveal normal cardiac enzymes, a cholesterol of 245 mg/dl and a normal blood count.

The chest x-ray is normal.

The patient's ECG is shown below:

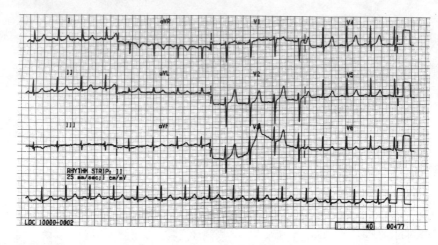

INTERPRETATION OF ECG: Normal.

QUESTIONS

1. What is the diagnosis?
2. What features differentiate this case from that of chronic stable angina?
3. What are the most accepted pathophysiologic mechanisms of this condition?
4. What are the initial steps in therapy?
5. If the patient continues to have unstable symptoms, what are the appropriate steps?

ANSWERS

1. Unstable angina. Other labels have been given to this condition, including preinfarction angina, crescendo angina, progressive coronary insufficiency, and angina decubitus. This suggests that unstable angina is not a single entity but rather a combination of syndromes.
2. The distinguishing characteristics of unstable angina are that it often occurs at rest or with minimal provocation, usually lasts longer, is less responsive to nitroglycerin, and is more often associated with ECG changes.
3. Although progression of atherosclerosis was thought to be the major factor in the past, more recent investigation suggests that coronary thrombosis, platelet aggregation and coronary artery spasm are frequent causes of unstable angina.
4. The patient should be hospitalized, sedated and observed with electrocardiographic monitoring. Nitrates, beta blockers and calcium blockers are the cornerstones of pharmacologic treatment. Goals of therapy ought to include aggressive treatment of any hypertension and keeping the pulse rate to 60. Aspirin is useful for its platelet-inhibiting effect. (The Veterans Administration study used 325 mg/day and showed a significant decrease in myocardial infarction and death in the aspirin group compared with the placebo group.) Most patients will stabilize with intensive medical therapy.
5. A small percentage of patients will remain unstable despite medical therapy. For this group, it is recommended to start intravenous nitroglycerin and place a balloon flotation catheter with the aim of keeping the wedge pressure below 15. If pain persists, an intra-aortic balloon pump should be placed, and the patient should be considered for angiography and, possibly, emergent angioplasty or bypass surgery.

PEARLS

1. Full-dose intravenous heparin has been shown to decrease the occurrence of acute MI in randomized studies and is used in many centers as an important part of therapy.
2. If the patient's symptoms are stabilized, there is generally no need to proceed emergently to coronary angiography. Prospective randomized

trials have shown no clear-cut advantage in comparing medical and medical-plus-surgical therapy in terms of morbidity or mortality.

## PITFALLS

1. Exercise testing should not be performed until the patient is stable or pain-free for over 24 hours. The presence of ECG changes of ischemia during angina often precludes the necessity of exercise testing.
2. Despite classic historical features of unstable angina, large groups (10-20%) of angiographically studied patients will show normal coronary arteries.

## REFERENCES

Faxon DP, Detre KM, McCabe CH, et al: Role of percutaneous transluminal coronary angioplasty in the treatment of unstable angina. Am J Cardiol 53:131C, 1984.

Lewis HD Jr, Davis JW, Archibald DG, et al: Protective effects of aspirin against acute myocardial infarction and death in men with unstable angina: Results of a Veterans Administration Cooperative Study. N Engl J Med 309:396, 1983.

Moise A, Theroux P, Talyams Y, et al: Unstable angina and progression of atherosclerosis. N Engl J Med 309:685, 1983.

Pepine CJ, Feldman RL, Hill JA, et al: Clinical outcome after treatment of rest angina with calcium blockers: Comparative experience during the initial year of therapy with diltiazem, nifedipine and verapamil. Am Heart J 106:1341, 1983.

## CASE 3: TRANSIENT ST ELEVATION

HISTORY

A 47-year-old cocktail waitress with severe chest pain which awakened her from sleep is brought to the emergency room at 3:00 a.m. by the paramedics. She has no previous cardiac history and takes no medications. She has a history of smoking but has no other risk factors for coronary artery disease.

EXAMINATION

On initial examination her blood pressure is 110/80; heart rate is 75, and respirations, 14. Her skin is pale and cool. Cardiac examination reveals a regular rhythm with occasional premature beats, S4 and no murmur.

HOSPITAL COURSE

An ECG obtained upon arrival is shown in Figure 1 below. The patient is given nitroglycerin for relief of the pain. A repeat ECG after pain relief is shown in Figure 2. Serial ECG's and enzymes over the next 48 hours reveal no myocardial injury. On her 3rd hospital day at 3:00 a.m. she has severe chest pain and suffers a cardiac arrest (Figure 3).

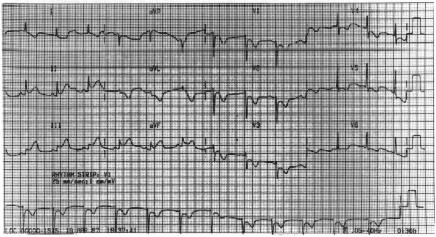

Figure 1

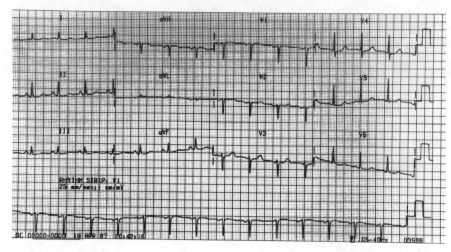

Figure 2

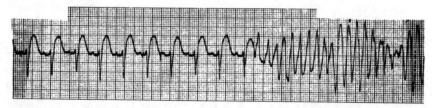

Figure 3

INTERPRETATION OF ECG's: Figure 1 shows marked ST elevation in the inferior leads and anterolateral ST depression and T wave inversion. In Figure 2 the ECG is normal except for inverted P waves in V1. Figure 3 shows sinus rhythm with ST elevation and the onset of ventricular fibrillation.

## QUESTIONS

1. What is the emergency management at the time of the arrest?
2. What is the clinical diagnosis?
3. Is it likely that the patient has fixed underlying coronary artery disease?
4. What is the initial pharmacologic management?
5. Should the patient have coronary angiography? Should ergonovine be given?

ANSWERS

1.  With defibrillation the patient returns immediately to sinus rhythm. After sublingual nitroglycerin her pain subsides and her ECG reverts to normal.
2.  Variant angina (Prinzmetal's angina, coronary artery spasm) is classically defined as a chest pain occurring typically at rest, usually associated with transient ST elevation, and usually responding to nitroglycerin. Often there is a circadian pattern to the clinical episodes of pain; the pain is usually not provoked by exercise. This syndrome may be associated with severe cardiac arrhythmia, acute myocardial infarction and sudden death.
3.  Most patients with variant angina have a demonstrable lesion in the coronary circulation, often in the artery or arteries at the site of spasm. Some cases (20%) will have no evidence of angiographic narrowing.
4.  Nitrates and calcium channel blockers are strongly indicated in this setting. Sublingual nitroglycerin and nitroglycerin spray are absorbed and usually relieve the spasm promptly (within seconds). The calcium channel blockers are also effective acutely and can be given sublingually.
5.  Cardiac catheterization is indicated. Dynamic constriction is seen in the affected artery or arteries if the patient has an episode of spasm at the time of the procedure. In this case, the clinical diagnosis of variant angina is clear-cut, so there is no reason to subject the patient to any potential morbidity with the spasm-inducing agent ergonovine. The use of ergonovine should be reserved for cases in which the diagnosis is unclear, and it should be administered in the catheterization laboratory where intracoronary nitroglycerin can be given to reverse the spasm.

PEARLS

1.  Most patients with variant angina will have fixed disease underlying the area of dynamic obstruction. Some patients have no fixed disease despite the obvious clinical picture of spasm.
2.  Patients with variant angina are often younger than patients with classic stable angina, and there is a lesser preponderance of males among variant angina patients than among stable angina patients.

3. Patients with variant angina and normal coronary angiograms are more likely to have pure nonexertional angina and ST elevation in the inferior leads, while patients with variant angina and obstructive lesions with spasm often have exertional angina and anterolateral ischemia.

## PITFALLS

1. Most, but not all, patients with coronary spasm have ST elevation. Some may have ST depression.
2. The response of patients with variant angina to beta blocker therapy is variable. There is theoretic reason to avoid beta blockers because the beta blockade may allow unopposed alpha receptor-mediated coronary constriction to occur.
3. Variant angina patients in whom myocardial ischemia is caused largely by spasm respond best to nitroglycerin and calcium blockers; beta blockers and coronary bypass surgery are of little, if any, value in this group.

## REFERENCES

Hillis TD, Braunwald E: Coronary artery spasm. N Engl J Med 299:695, 1978.

Oliva PB, Potts DE, Pluss RG: Coronary arterial spasm in Prinzmetal angina: Documentation by coronary arteriography. N Engl J Med 288:745, 1973.

Prinzmetal M, Kennamer R, Merliss R, et al: Angina pectoris: A variant form of angina pectoris. Am J Med 27:375, 1959.

Stein JH, Ambrose JA, King BD, Herman MV: An integrated approach to the recognition and treatment of variant angina. Cardiovasc Rev Rep 3:1297, 1982.

## CASE 4: HYPOTENSION AND INFERIOR INFARCTION

HISTORY

A 58-year-old insurance salesman is admitted with several hours of substernal chest pressure with nausea, vomiting, diaphoresis and lightheadedness. He denies any previous history of chest discomfort or known heart disease. His risk factors for coronary artery disease include cigarette smoking and a family history of premature myocardial infarction.

EXAMINATION

Blood pressure is 86 and palpable; pulse is thready at 88/minute. He is pale, diaphoretic and lethargic. The jugular veins are distended. The lungs are clear without rales or wheezes. The heart sounds are normal, and there is a 4th heart sound appreciated at the lower left sternal border. There are no murmurs, and the remainder of the examination is normal.

ADDITIONAL DATA

The chest x-ray is normal.

The standard 12-lead ECG plus additional right precordial leads V3R and V4R are shown below:

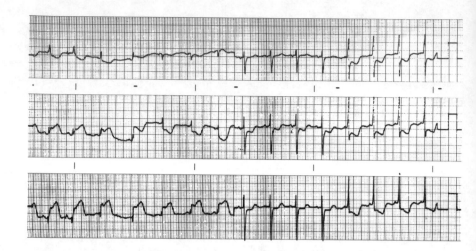

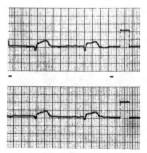

INTERPRETATION OF ECG:   Acute ST elevation in the inferior leads; anterolateral ST depression and T wave inversion.   The right precordial leads show ST elevation.

CLUE FROM THE HISTORY AND EXAMINATION

This man presents with arterial hypotension (and hypoperfusion) in the setting of an acute inferior wall myocardial infarction; the jugular venous pressure is elevated, yet the lungs are clear, suggesting right heart dysfunction without left-sided failure.

## QUESTIONS

1. What is the likely explanation for these clinical findings?
2. What diagnostic procedure is indicated?
3. What is the appropriate treatment for hypotension in this setting?
4. What noninvasive studies might confirm the diagnosis?

ANSWERS

1. Right ventricular (RV) infarction commonly presents with arterial hypotension, elevated jugular pressure and clear lung fields in the setting of an inferior wall myocardial infarction.
2. Hypotension with signs of hypoperfusion in the setting of an acute myocardial infarction is an appropriate indication for right heart catheterization at the bedside with a balloon-directed pulmonary artery catheter. The findings of elevated right heart filling pressures (with minimal elevation in the pulmonary capillary wedge pressure) will confirm the diagnosis of hemodynamically significant RV infarction, and serial hemodynamic measurements will help facilitate therapy.
3. Vigorous fluid therapy will increase right-sided output and thus improve left-sided preload and cardiac output; inotropic support should only be added after the pulmonary capillary wedge pressure has been optimized.
4. A gated blood pool scan (MUGA) may show abnormal RV wall motion and dilatation out of proportion to left-sided dysfunction. In addition, the technetium pyrophosphate ("hot-spot") scan may show abnormal uptake in the area of the right ventricle after 48-72 hours following the infarction. A 2-dimensional echocardiogram can demonstrate RV enlargement and dysfunction.

PEARLS

1. Some elements of RV infarction have been demonstrated pathologically in up to 1/3 of inferior wall infarctions; however, it only achieves clinical relevance in 1-2% of inferior infarcts.
2. Shock due to RV infarction represents a favorable subset of cardiogenic shock with a better than 50% survival, compared with the 10-15% survival in patients with shock accompanying anterior wall infarction.
3. Elevation of the ST segment in the right-sided precordial lead V4R is a useful electrocardiographic clue to the presence of RV infarction.
4. Isolated infarction of the free wall of the right ventricle is rare because of the dual blood supply from the branches of the right coronary artery and from the RV branches of the left anterior descending artery.

## PITFALLS

1. Hypotension due to excessive vagal outflow may occur in the setting of acute myocardial infarction and initially mimic shock due to left or right ventricular infarction.
2. Elevated right atrial, RV end-diastolic and pulmonary artery diastolic pressures may equal pulmonary capillary wedge pressure in patients with RV infarction; this hemodynamic finding may be identical to that in patients with pericardial constriction.
3. Initial hemodynamic measurements may be nondiagnostic in patients with RV infarction who are volume depleted because of low intake, vomiting or excessive diaphoresis; fluid loading may be required to demonstrate the characteristic elevation of right-sided pressures in these patients.

## REFERENCES

Baigrie RS, Haq A, Morgan CD, et al: The spectrum of right ventricular involvement in inferior wall myocardial infarction: A clinical, hemodynamic and noninvasive study. J Am Coll Cardiol 1:1396, 1983.

Candell-Riera J, Figueras J, Valle V, et al: Right ventricular infarction: Relationships between ST segment elevation in V4R and hemodynamic, scintigraphic and echocardiographic findings in patients with acute inferior myocardial infarction. Am Heart J 101:281, 1981.

Cohn JN: Right ventricular infarction revisited. Am J Cardiol 43:666, 1979.

Isner JM, Roberts WC: Right ventricular infarction complicating left ventricular infarction secondary to coronary heart disease. Am J Cardiol 42:885, 1978.

Lopez-Sendon J, Coma-Canella I, Gamallo C: Sensitivity and specificity of hemodynamic criteria in the diagnosis of acute right ventricular infarction. Circulation 64:515, 1981.

Sharpe DN, Botvinick EH, Shames DM, et al: The noninvasive diagnosis of right ventricular infarction. Circulation 57:483, 1978.

## CASE 5: NEW MURMUR FOLLOWING MYOCARDIAL INFARCTION

HISTORY

A 71-year-old woman presents with 8 hours of increasing substernal chest pressure radiating to the left arm, shortness of breath, and diaphoresis.

EXAMINATION

Examination on admission reveals an alert, elderly woman in moderate discomfort without respiratory distress. Her blood pressure is 146/78; her pulse is 108 and regular. There are bibasilar crackles, and the heart reveals apical dyskinesis to palpation with a prominent 4th heart sound. No murmurs or rubs are appreciated.

The admitting ECG is shown below:

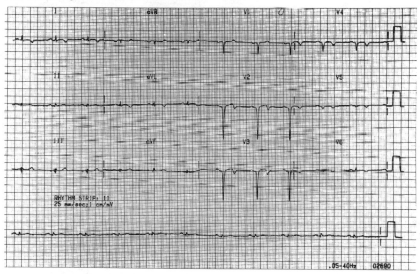

INTERPRETATION OF ECG: Anterolateral myocardial infarction with ST-T wave changes.

HOSPITAL COURSE

The patient is treated with morphine sulfate, topical nitroglycerin, oxygen and furosemide, with improvement in her pain over the next few hours. Serial ECG's confirm an anterior infarction, and creatine kinase (CK) peaked at 1220 total (normal, 0-145) with an MB fraction of 22%. She is without further chest discomfort or signs of congestive heart failure.

On the 4th hospital day you are called to see the patient because she is confused and in moderate distress, with a heart rate of 136 and blood pressure of 90/46. On your examination there is no audible or palpable pulsus paradoxus. New jugular venous distension to the angle of the jaw with the patient at 45 degrees is apparent. The lungs reveal diffuse crackles and mild expiratory wheezing. There is a thrill palpable at the lower left sternal border, with a IV/VI systolic murmur radiating to the lower right and left sternal borders.

An ECG shows additional nonspecific ST and T wave changes and sinus tachycardia but is otherwise unchanged.

CLUE FROM THE HISTORY AND EXAMINATION

This elderly woman develops sudden and dramatic deterioration several days after an anterior MI. Although severe global ischemia or extension of infarction could theoretically produce this clinical picture, the murmur and thrill are indicative of a mechanical complication of acute MI.

QUESTIONS

1. What possible diagnoses need to be considered when one suspects a mechanical complication of MI?
2. What diagnostic tests are indicated?
3. What immediate therapeutic interventions should be instituted?
4. What is this patient's prognosis with medical therapy, as compared with surgical therapy?

ANSWERS

1. Mechanical complications of acute MI include ventricular septal defect (VSD), rupture of the left ventricular (LV) free wall, and papillary muscle dysfunction. A new loud holosystolic murmur may be present either with a VSD or with severe mitral regurgitation secondary to papillary muscle dysfunction. The presence of the thrill several days following infarction of the anterior wall of the heart is characteristic of a post infarction VSD.

2. Prompt right heart catheterization with a Swan-Ganz catheter is indicated. Specifically, findings of a step-up in the oxygen saturation from the right atrium to the right ventricle or pulmonary artery of 10% or greater is indicative of a left-to-right shunt, such as with a VSD. Echocardiography may show the VSD directly, or the injection of agitated saline "contrast" into a peripheral vein may demonstrate shunting through a VSD. Doppler technique may delineate abnormal flow in the right ventricle.

3. Initial therapy to stabilize this patient should include aggressive (systemic) afterload reduction with intravenous sodium nitroprusside in an attempt to increase forward flow from the left ventricle and decrease left-to-right shunting. The intra-aortic balloon pump (IABP), which mechanically unloads the left ventricle and yet maintains coronary perfusion pressure during diastole, has been exceedingly useful in temporarily stabilizing these patients.

4. Post infarction VSD is associated with an extremely poor outcome (a mortality rate of 25% in the first 24 hours and 90% in the first 2 months) with medical management alone. Aggressive surgical repair has been associated with an overall survival of greater than 50% and is excellent (more than 80%) in patients who can be stabilized and undergo surgery more than 3 weeks following the infarction.

PEARLS

1. Mechanical complications of MI generally occur 3-6 days following infarction, when the myocardium is the weakest.

2. A post necrotic VSD occurs in up to 2% of patients admitted to the coronary care unit with acute infarction.

3. Risk factors that are associated with this complication of MI include age greater than 70, female sex, hypertension and LV hypertrophy.

4. Sixty percent of postinfarction VSD's accompany anterior infarctions and are often associated with single-vessel coronary artery disease.
5. VSD's that complicate inferior MI's are commonly associated with 3-vessel coronary artery disease, and mortality is higher with these than with VSD's accompanying anterior infarctions.
6. The ratio of pulmonary to systemic blood flow (Qp/Qs), and thus the amount of left-to-right shunting, can be estimated by measurement of oxygen saturations (satn) at the time of right heart catheterization:

$$Qp/Qs = \frac{(Aortic\ O_2\ satn) - (Right\ atrial\ O_2\ satn)}{(Left\ atrial\ O_2\ satn) - (Pulm\ artery\ O_2\ satn)}$$

PITFALLS

1. Hemodynamic deterioration occurs in the majority of patients with a VSD following acute MI, and in only 20-25% can surgery be delayed to 6 weeks following infarction.
2. A decrease in the intensity of the murmur and in the estimated Qp/Qs may occur with treatment. This may be a sign of response to therapy; however, it may also be secondary to rising right-sided pressures due to right heart failure with narrowing of the pressure gradient across the large defect.

REFERENCES

Brandt B III, Wright CB, Ehrenhaft JL: Ventricular septal defect following myocardial infarction. Ann Thorac Surg 27:580, 1979.
Daggett WM, Guyton RA, Mundth ED, et al: Surgery for post-myocardial infarct ventricular septal defect. Ann Surg 186:260, 1979.
Gold HK, Leinbach RC, Sanders CA, et al: Intra-aortic balloon pumping for ventricular septal defect or mitral regurgitation complicating acute myocardial infarction. Circulation 47:1191, 1973.
Labovitz AJ, Miller LW, Kennedy HL: Mechanical complications of acute myocardial infarction. Cardiovasc Rev Rep 5:948, 1984.
Miller DC, Stinson EB: Surgical management of acute mechanical defects secondary to myocardial infarction. Am J Surg 141:677, 1981.

## CASE 6: ACUTE MYOCARDIAL INFARCTION WITH BUNDLE BRANCH BLOCK

HISTORY

A 48-year-old man comes to the emergency room with 6 hours of anterior chest pressure and lightheadedness. He has never had this type of discomfort before but has had exertional aching in his left shoulder and arm over the last few months. He smokes 1 1/2 packs of cigarettes daily and has had high blood pressure for 10 years. He had a checkup 6 months ago and was told "everything was okay," including his electrocardiogram.

EXAMINATION

The patient is pale and diaphoretic, in no respiratory distress. His blood pressure is 160/95; his heart rate is 100 and regular. The lungs are clear, and the carotid volume is normal. There is a loud 4th heart sound, and no murmur or S3.

CLUE FROM THE ECG

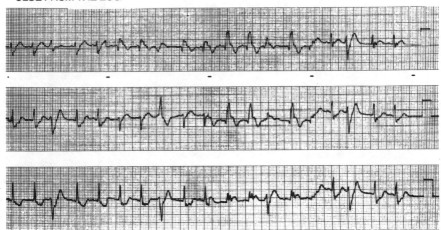

QUESTIONS

1. What is the diagnosis suggested by the history and ECG?
2. What is the significance of the intraventricular conduction delay?
3. What is the likelihood that this man will develop congestive heart failure (CHF) or complete heart block (CHB)?
4. Is a temporary pacemaker indicated?
5. When would you recommend a permanent pacemaker for a patient after an acute myocardial infarction?

ANSWERS

1. The prolonged chest pressure and the elevated ST segments in V1-V3 of the ECG are indicative of acute anterior myocardial infarction (MI). The ECG also shows right bundle branch block (RBBB), sinus tachycardia with premature ventricular contractions, and diffuse ST-T wave changes.
2. The intraventricular conduction delay in the setting of acute MI is associated with increased mortality and morbidity (CHF and heart block) due to greater pump dysfunction and electrical instability.
3. RBBB in acute MI progresses to CHB in an average of 20-30% of cases; significant CHF, as evidenced by pulmonary edema or cardiogenic shock, is seen in over 40% of cases.
4. In this patient with RBBB alone, the indication for temporary pacing is controversial. Most authors recommend temporary pacing for patients at highest risk for progression to CHB; these include patients with alternating right and left bundle branch block (BBB) and patients with bifascicular block, i.e., RBBB and either left anterior superior hemiblock (LASH) or left posterior inferior hemiblock (LPIH).
5. Permanent pacemakers have been shown to improve survival and are thus indicated in patients with bifascicular block in acute MI who evidence transient Mobitz type II AV block or CHB.

PEARLS

1. Some form of intraventricular conduction delay complicates approximately 20% of cases of acute MI; bundle branch block or bifascicular block accounts for over 1/2 of these cases.
2. Bundle branch block occurs more commonly with anterior MI than with inferior or lateral infarction; 75% of infarctions with bundle branch block that can be localized involve the anterior wall.
3. The overall mortality of acute MI with BBB is 20-30%, as compared with 10-15% when infarction is not associated with this complication.
4. Left anterior superior hemiblock (LASH) is the intraventricular conduction defect (IVCD) most commonly seen with MI; right bundle branch block with LASH is the next most common.
5. First degree AV block and Wenckebach-type 2nd degree heart block are not associated with increased risk in the peri-infarction period.
6. Over 75% of deaths in patients with acute MI complicated by bundle

branch block are due to congestive heart failure; fewer than 10% are due to abrupt complete heart block.

PITFALLS

1. Although temporary pacemakers are recommended when bifascicular block complicates acute anterior MI, there is no proven increase in survival in these patients.
2. Approximately 1/3 of patients with BBB who develop 3rd degree (complete) heart block do so without warning periods of intermittent (2nd degree) block.
3. Mortality from acute MI with BBB is further increased in patients who have sustained a previous infarction.

REFERENCES

Domenighetti G, Perret C: Intraventricular conduction disturbances in acute myocardial infarction: Short and long-term prognosis. Eur J Cardiol 11:51, 1980.
Hindman MC, Wagner GS, JaRo M, et al: The clinical significance of bundle branch block complicating acute myocardial infarction: 1. Clinical characteristics, hospital mortality, and one-year follow-up. Circulation 58:679, 1978.
Hindman MC, Wagner GS, JaRo M, et al: The clinical significance of bundle branch block complicating acute myocardial infarction: 2. Indications for temporary and permanent pacemaker insertion. Circulation 58:689, 1978.
Jacobson LB, Lester RM, Scheinman MM: Management of acute bundle branch block and bradyarrhythmias. Med Clin North Am 63:93, 1979.
Klein RC, Vera Z, Mason DT: Intraventricular conduction defects in acute myocardial infarction: Incidence, prognosis, and therapy. Am Heart J 108:1007, 1984.

## CASE 7: PROLONGED CHEST PAIN

HISTORY

A 58-year-old white man is admitted to the hospital with a chief complaint of intense retrosternal pressure and aching discomfort of 6 hours duration. He was awakened at 4:00 a.m., and the initial pain was accompanied by nausea with attempted emesis and diaphoresis but no shortness of breath. There is no prior cardiac history, but he describes a decline in exercise tolerance due to weakness and fatigue. He has had occasional exertional epigastric and neck discomfort, especially after eating. He has not had orthopnea, dyspnea or edema. Risk factors for coronary disease include 50 pack years of smoking and a family history of atherosclerosis, with his father having died suddenly at the age of 48. He takes no medications and denies palpitations or syncope. During the examination his pain subsided.

EXAMINATION

Examination reveals a blood pressure of 108/60 and a heart rate of 50 and regular. He is alert, diaphoretic and pale. The lungs are clear, and cardiovascular examination shows a jugular venous pressure of 7 cm of H2O. The left ventricular impulse is not palpable; there is a prominent S4 and no murmur. The abdomen is benign, and peripheral pulses are intact.

CLUE FROM THE ECG

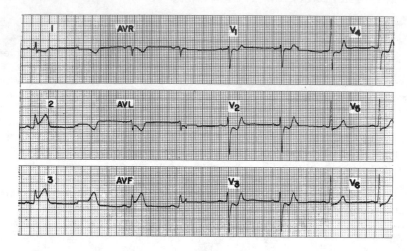

INTERPRETATION OF ECG: Sinus bradycardia; hyperacute inferior ST elevation; ST depression in I, aVL, and V1-V4.

QUESTIONS

1. Does the bradycardia require treatment, and what is appropriate?
2. What is the location of this acute infarction, and which coronary artery (arteries) might be involved?
3. What is the pathophysiologic event involved with acute infarction?
4. Is right ventricular infarction present here?
5. Should acute intervention with streptokinase or percutaneous transluminal coronary angioplasty be attempted?
6. What percentage of patients with acute myocardial infarction have an S4 gallop on initial physical examination?

ANSWERS

1.  No. Treatment is not required because the patient is not hypotensive
    or symptomatic. Transient autonomic disturbances occur commonly in
    acute MI, with parasympathetic overactivity (bradycardia and
    hypotension) predominating in patients with acute inferior
    infarctions. Temporary pacemaker insertion with an inferior MI is
    usually not required, since the level of block is at the AV node, is
    usually transient, and often responds to therapy with atropine and
    fluid challenge.

2.  ST elevation in leads II, III and AVF is indicative of acute inferior MI.
    This is most commonly due to right coronary artery occlusion. In
    some cases inferior MI is the result of occlusion of the circumflex
    coronary artery.

3.  In the majority of patients, coronary thrombus formation at the site
    of an atherosclerotic plaque is responsible for the acute occlusion of
    the infarct-related artery.

4.  The available data do not allow a firm conclusion about this; however,
    it is a question to be asked with every inferior MI. The diagnostic
    study of choice is acute application of the right precordial leads (V3R
    and V4R). Hypotension and jugular venous distension in the absence of
    signs of LV failure are the clinical bedside clues of RV infarction and
    are not present in this case. ST elevation in V1 or in the right
    precordial leads (V3R and V4R) is a useful clue and should be looked
    for in all inferior MI's.

5.  Although there is no dogmatic answer to this question, most protocols
    for such intervention require initiation of therapy within 4 hours.
    Since the patient has been symptomatic for 6 hours, little or no
    benefit would be expected from this approach. Additionally, several
    studies have revealed that patients with inferior MI--in
    contradistinction to those with anterior MI--derive minimal or no
    survival advantage from thrombolytic therapy.

6.  A 4th heart sound (S4 or atrial gallop), which is a sign of decreased
    ventricular compliance, is the most consistent abnormal finding in
    acute MI. With careful auscultation an S4 will be present in virtually
    all patients with acute MI.

PEARLS

1.  Although controversial, use of prophylactic lidocaine can be supported in most patients, because 50% of patients who suffer ventricular fibrillation show no "warning" dysrhythmias. Because of a higher incidence of toxicity in the elderly, lidocaine should be used with caution or avoided in this group.
2.  The severity of pain is not closely related to the extent of myocardial necrosis.
3.  Creatine kinase (CK) isoenzymes normally peak at approximately 24 hours and usually don't become positive until 4-6 hours after the onset of symptoms. The historical evaluation and ECG remain the primary tools for diagnosis in the acute phase.
4.  Routine laboratory studies often show a mild increase of blood sugar and leukocytosis in response to the stress of the infarct.

PITFALLS

1.  The insertion of a temporary pacer should be avoided in the often transient and asymptomatic bradycardia of acute inferior MI.
2.  At times, symptoms of acute inferior MI are limited to nausea, emesis and epigastric or low retrosternal discomfort, and the clinician must keep a high index of suspicion for acute ischemia.

REFERENCES

Alpert JA, Braunwald E:  Pathological and clinical manifestations of acute myocardial infarction.  In Braunwald E (ed):  Heart Disease:  A Textbook of Cardiovascular Medicine.  Philadelphia, WB Saunders, 1980, p 1309.
DeWood MA, Spores J, Notske R, et al:  Prevalence of total coronary occlusion during the early hours of transmural myocardial infarction. N Engl J Med 303:897, 1980.
Hancock EW:  Ischemic heart disease:  Acute myocardial infarction.  In Rubenstein E, Federman DD (eds):  Scientific American Medicine.  New York, Scientific American, 1982, ch 10, p 1.
Hurst JW, Kug SB, Kriesinger GC, et al:  Atherosclerotic coronary heart disease:  Recognition, prognosis and treatment.  In Hurst JW (ed.):  The Heart.  New York, McGraw-Hill, 1986, p 973.

Kent KM, Smith ER, Redwood DR, et al:   Electrical stability of acutely ischemic myocardium:   Influences of heart rate and vagal stimulation. Circulation 47:291, 1973.

## CASE 8: CHEST PAIN WITH PERSISTENT ST AND T WAVE CHANGES

CLINICAL PRESENTATION

A 68-year-old meat packer presents with 20 minutes of substernal chest heaviness associated with some diaphoresis and no nausea. One year ago the patient was admitted for chest pain, and a myocardial infarction (MI) was ruled out. The patient has risk factors of smoking and a positive family history of coronary artery disease.

ADDITIONAL DATA

Serial enzymes show a mild rise in creatine kinase (CK) with MB fraction of 18%.

The ECG, shown below, remains unchanged over 24 hours:

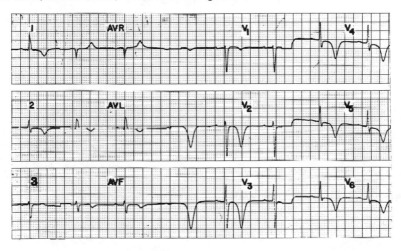

INTERPRETATION OF ECG: T wave inversion V1-V5 compatible with ischemia or infarction.

QUESTIONS

1. What is the diagnosis?
2. What is the likelihood that the patient will have a transmural MI in the next year?
3. What coronary artery is probably involved in this setting? Is there likely to be viable myocardium in the area of the infarct?
4. What are the treatment implications for this condition?

ANSWERS

1. Nontransmural myocardial infarction (NTMI). NTMI is also called subendocardial infarction or a non-Q wave infarction. This is defined as a clinical syndrome of typical pain, abnormalities in enzymes, and persistent ECG changes limited to ST segments and T waves.
2. Natural history studies show that the reinfarction rate is high in this setting and occurs in approximately 1/4-1/3 of cases within the next year.
3. The left anterior descending coronary artery is likely to be involved. Often there is viable but jeopardized myocardium at a high risk of reinfarction.
4. Because the patient with an NIMI has a potentially unstable condition, a more aggressive diagnostic and therapeutic approach is warranted. Early cardiac catheterization with possible revascularization with percutaneous transluminal coronary angioplasty (PTCA) or coronary artery bypass surgery (CABG) is suggested.

PEARLS

1. The extent and severity of coronary artery disease is similar for transmural and nontransmural MI patients.
2. There is a higher incidence of complete occlusion in the artery supplying the affected area of the infarct in transmural MI patients. The nontransmural MI patients often have a highly stenotic but patent coronary artery and a higher incidence of collaterals.

PITFALLS

1. Nontransmural MI is diagnosed on the basis of the lack of Q waves on the ECG. The assumption has been made that ECG-defined NTMI predicts that only the subendocardium is involved. There is, at times, a discrepancy between the extent of infarction defined by the ECG and that noted pathologically. For instance, a very small subendocardial MI documented pathologically may cause Q waves. Although the electrographic definition does not predict the anatomic extent of infarction, the distinction between nontransmural and transmural infarction still appears to be clinically worthwhile.
2. The patient with a non-Q wave infarct is often perceived as having a "benign" process. This is a mistaken notion. The natural history of a

high preponderance of repeated infarct in the ensuing year (25% of patients) and the often viable but ischemic myocardium at risk should alert the clinician that this is a potentially unstable condition.

## REFERENCES

Cheitlin MD:  Nontransmural and transmural MI:  Important clinical differences?  J Cardiovasc Med 9:471, 1984.

Hutter AM, DeSanctis RW, Flynn T, Yeatman LA:  Nontransmural myocardial infarction:  A comparison of hospital and late clinical course of patients with that of matched patients with transmural anterior and inferior myocardial infarction.  Am J Cardiol 48:595, 1981.

Mormor A, Sobel BE, Roberts R:  Factors presaging early recurrent myocardial infarction ("extension").  Am J Cardiol 48:603, 1981.

## CASE 9: EARLY PRESENTATION OF CHEST PAIN

HISTORY

A 54-year-old physician comes to the emergency room from his office across the street; he has experienced increasing chest pressure and diaphoresis for 45 minutes. Over the past 2 days he has had 2 mild episodes of this discomfort and has felt more tired than usual. There is no history of heart disease, but he was a heavy smoker until 1 year ago and has had long-standing hypertension currently controlled on medications. He denies significant previous illness except for a duodenal ulcer 3 years ago.

EXAMINATION

An anxious, pale middle-aged man with blood pressure of 154/90 and heart rate of 84. There is no jugular venous distension, and the carotid pulsations are normal. The lungs reveal basilar crackles, and there is an S4 gallop. The remainder of the examination is normal.

ADDITIONAL DATA

The ECG is shown below. Sublingual nitroglycerin and sublingual nifedipine do not improve the discomfort or change the ECG.

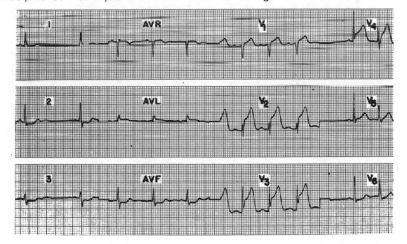

INTERPRETATION OF ECG: Hyperacute anterior ST elevation compatible with acute infarction; there is a sinus pause and a junctional escape beat.

QUESTIONS

1. What is the diagnosis from the history and ECG?
2. What is the likelihood that there is a complete occlusion of the left anterior descending coronary artery?
3. What might be considered to limit the size of this impending myocardial infarction?
4. What are contraindications for thrombolytic therapy?
5. What are common signs that reperfusion has been achieved?
6. Will this patient develop a myocardial infarction by ECG and enzyme criteria, even if reperfusion occurs?

ANSWERS

1. The history and ECG are compatible with an acute anteroseptal myocardial infarction (MI).

2. Patients presenting within the first 4 hours of an MI with ST segment elevation have complete occlusion of the infarct-related artery in nearly 90% of cases. In this patient, with ST segment elevation in the anterior precordial leads, the likelihood of complete occlusion of the left anterior descending artery is high.

3. The most promising method of limiting infarct size and thus preserving left ventricular function is acute reperfusion to the area of infarction. Reperfusion techniques include thrombolytic therapy (intravenous or intracoronary), percutaneous transluminal coronary angioplasty (PTCA), and emergency coronary artery bypass grafting (CABG). Intravenous thrombolytic therapy does not require cardiac catheterization and has the advantage of potentially providing earlier reperfusion in the setting of acute infarction.

4. Absolute contraindications are active internal hemorrhage or prior cerebrovascular disease (or procedure) within the past 2 months. Relative contraindications to the use of thrombolytic therapy include conditions predisposing to bleeding, such as recent major surgery, uncontrolled hypertension, cardiopulmonary resuscitation with rib fracture, and puncture of a noncompressible blood vessel. In addition, advanced age is associated with a higher incidence of bleeding complications.

5. It is common following successful thrombolysis to see significant reduction in pain with return of ST segments toward baseline. Ventricular arrhythmias, including frequent PVC's, idioventricular rhythm and ventricular tachycardia, are characteristic "reperfusion arrhythmias." In addition, creatine kinase levels often show an early peak (at or before 12 hours) when reperfusion has occurred. Without angiographic proof of recanalization, these ECG changes, arrhythmias and characteristic enzyme patterns are only inferential evidence of reperfusion.

6. Nearly all patients with 30-45 minutes of ischemic pain and ST segment elevation will have electrocardiographic and enzymatic evidence of myocardial necrosis, even with clinically evident reperfusion. It is often difficult to assess whether there has been significant salvage of jeopardized myocardium.

PEARLS

1. It is suggested by recent studies that treatment with thrombolytic agents should begin within 4 hours of the onset of symptoms for there to be a demonstrable effect on infarct size and left ventricular function. This is a guideline rather than a dogmatic rule.
2. Treatment with intravenous (or intracoronary) streptokinase or urokinase is associated with the production of a "systemic lytic state" with marked decreases in fibrinogen levels and abnormalities in all tests of coagulation.
3. Clinical trials have shown that "clot-specific" thrombolytic agents administered intravenously (e.g., recombinant tissue-type plasminogen activator) are nearly twice as effective as intravenous streptokinase in achieving thrombolysis.

PITFALLS

1. Although therapy with intravenous streptokinase may be undertaken with less delay and expense and without the need of a cardiac catheterization laboratory, intravenous streptokinase is less efficacious than streptokinase infused directly into the infarct-related artery.
2. It remains unclear what is the optimal therapy for patients who have undergone thrombolytic therapy; long-term treatment options include oral anticoagulation, angioplasty and bypass surgery. Of these, angioplasty has been shown in many cases to be particularly beneficial.
3. Several studies are pointing to improved survival, acutely and in the 1st year, with successful thrombolysis. The most dramatic reduction in mortality appears to be in that subset of patients who receive lytic therapy within 1 hour of the onset of pain.

REFERENCES

Braunwald E: The aggressive treatment of acute myocardial infarction. Circulation 71:1087, 1985.
DeWood MA, Spores J, Notske R, et al: Prevalence of total coronary occlusion during the early hours of transmural myocardial infarction. N Engl J Med 303:897, 1980.

GISSI Study: Effectiveness of intravenous thrombolytic treatment in acute myocardial infarction. Lancet I:397, 1986.

Koren G, Weiss AT, Hasin Y, et al: Prevention of myocardial damage in acute myocardial ischemia by early treatment with intravenous streptokinase. N Engl J Med 313:1384, 1985.

Laffel GL, Braunwald E: Thrombolytic therapy: A new strategy for the treatment of acute myocardial infarction: Parts I and II. N Engl J Med 311:710, 770, 1984.

Mathey DG, Heehan FH, Schofer J, et al: Time from onset of symptoms to thrombolytic therapy: A major determinant of myocardial salvage in patients with acute transmural infarction. J Am Coll Cardiol 6:518, 1985.

Rentrop KP: Thrombolytic therapy in patients with acute myocardial infarction. Circulation 71:627, 1985.

Simoons ML, Serruys PW, Brand M, et al: Improved survival after early thrombolysis in acute myocardial infarction. Lancet II:578, 1985.

TIMI Study Group: The thrombolysis in myocardial infarction (TIMI) trial: Phase 1 findings. N Engl J Med 312:932, 1985.

## CASE 10: YOUNG BOY WITH FEVER, ARTHRALGIAS AND A NEW HEART MURMUR

HISTORY

A 7-year-old Vietnamese boy is brought to the clinic because of fever and joint swelling of 2 weeks duration. The inflammation began in his right knee and then involved his left knee, elbows and right ankle in succession. He has had fever to as high as 38.3oC. There is no history of recent sore throat, skin rash or cardiorespiratory symptoms. He and his family immigrated to this country 3 weeks ago; no one else in the family has similar symptoms.

EXAMINATION

A thin, well-developed boy appearing mildly ill. His blood pressure is 110/66; heart rate is 92 and regular; temperature is 38oC. There is warmth and tenderness of the right ankle and right elbow with full range of motion. The skin is clear; however, there are several small, nontender nodules over the extensor tendons of the fingers on both hands. The pharynx is benign, and the carotid upstroke and volume are normal. The precordial impulse is normal to palpation. There is a grade III/VI apical murmur that is holosystolic and blowing in quality. There is also a short II/VI diastolic murmur at the apex following a 3rd heart sound. The neurologic examination is normal.

ADDITIONAL DATA

The ECG shows 1st degree AV block. The chest radiograph is normal.

CLUE FROM THE HISTORY AND EXAMINATION

This boy, recently from Southeast Asia, presents with the constellation of migratory arthritis, fever, subcutaneous nodules and heart murmurs. The pure, blowing quality of the systolic murmur and the presence of an apical diastolic murmur are strong evidence for organic heart disease.

QUESTIONS

1. What laboratory test(s) would help confirm the diagnosis?
2. What is the pathophysiology of this disease?
3. What is the most common neurologic disorder associated with this illness?
4. How does the carditis present?
5. What is the likelihood of this boy developing valvular heart disease following this acute episode?
6. What treatment would you institute?

ANSWERS

1.  In this patient, a positive throat culture for group A, beta-hemolytic streptococci or the presence of antistreptococcal antibodies in the serum (antistreptolysin O or antiDNAse B) would indicate recent streptococcal infection and confirm the diagnosis of acute rheumatic fever (ARF).
2.  Rheumatic fever is a postinfectious complication that follows streptococcal pharyngitis (not impetigo) caused by a rheumatogenic strain that is of sufficient duration and occurs in a susceptible host. The relative roles of humoral and cellular immunity and the importance of the cross-reactivity between human and streptococcal antigens remain controvorsial.
3.  Sydenham's chorea (St. Vitus' dance), which often occurs late in the course of rheumatic fever, is characterized by erratic and purposeless movements and personality changes, including emotional lability.
4.  The 4 manifestations of acute rheumatic carditis are: new organic murmurs, pericarditis or effusion, cardiomegaly with or without congestive heart failure, and arrhythmias such as nodal rhythms or heart block.
5.  The development and severity of chronic rheumatic heart disease is related to the degree of acute carditis. This patient, with apparently mild carditis, has only a small chance of developing severe rheumatic valvular disease if his carditis clears promptly and recurrences of rheumatic fever are prevented.
6.  In addition to bed rest and general supportive care, treatment should include: (1) eradication of the streptococcal organism with 10 days of intramuscular procaine penicillin or a single injection of benzathine penicillin; (2) anti-inflammatory treatment with salicylates, or corticosteroids with moderate or severe carditis; (3) secondary prevention of streptococcal infection and rheumatic fever with monthly benzathine penicillin or daily oral antibiotics; and (4) prevention of bacterial endocarditis with antibiotics prior to dental and other procedures associated with bacteremia.

PEARLS

1.  The incidence of acute rheumatic fever is relatively constant and averages 1-3% of cases of untreated exudative pharyngitis.

2. Recurrences of acute rheumatic fever are particularly high during the first few years following the initial episode and occur in as many as 20% of individuals who develop recurrent streptococcal pharyngitis.
3. Human lymphocyte antigen (HLA) B-883 appears to be associated with increased susceptibility to rheumatic fever. Nearly 75% of individuals with rheumatic fever are HLA B-883 positive, as compared to approximately 15% of the general population.
4. First degree AV block is common in acute rheumatic carditis; that the PR interval normalizes with atropine suggests this is a functional (and not structural) abnormality.
5. The revised Jones Criteria for the diagnosis of rheumatic fever consist of major and minor manifestations; the 5 major manifestations are: carditis, polyarthritis, chorea, erythema marginatum and subcutaneous nodules.

PITFALLS

1. Up to 50% of patients with rheumatic heart disease do not have a history of recognized acute rheumatic fever.
2. The preceding streptococcal pharyngitis can be nearly asymptomatic, and approximately 1/3 of patients with ARF do not recall "strep throat."
3. Antistreptolysin O (ASO) titers may be normal if the diagnosis of ARF is not made in the first 2 months. This occurs in patients who present with isolated (late) chorea or with chronic rheumatic carditis.
4. The titer of the ASO antibody is not indicative of disease activity or prognosis in ARF.

REFERENCES

Patarroyo M: Pathogenesis and immunogenetics of rheumatic fever. Semin Arthritis Rheum 13:102, 1983.
Stollerman GH: Rheumatic and heritable connective tissue diseases of the cardiovascular system. In Braunwald E (ed): Heart Disease. A Textbook of Cardiovascular Medicine. Philadelphia, WB Saunders, 1984, pp 1641-1656.
Williams RC Jr: Host factors in rheumatic fever and heart disease. Hosp Pract (August):125, 1982.

Zabriskie JB: Rheumatic fever: The interplay between host, genetics, and microbe: Lewis A. Conner Memorial Lecture. Circulation 71:1077, 1985.

## CASE 11: FEVER AND CHANGING HEART MURMUR

HISTORY

A 59-year-old woman is admitted with 2 weeks of fever and 3 days of increasing shortness of breath. Her physician first noted a grade II/VI systolic murmur several years previously. There is no history of rheumatic fever, chest pain, palpitations or congestive heart failure. She had routine teeth cleaning 4 weeks prior to the onset of her symptoms.

EXAMINATION

An acutely ill female in mild respiratory distress. Her temperature is 380C; heart rate is 112 and regular; blood pressure is 136/72; respiratory rate is 24. HEENT: Several conjunctival petechiae. The neck is supple without adenopathy and with normal jugular venous pulsations. The carotid upstroke and volume are normal. There are rales 1/3 of the way up bilaterally with mild expiratory wheezing. The left ventricular impulse is hyperdynamic and palpable in the 6th intercostal space 2 cm left of the midclavicular line. There is a summation gallop heard with the bell of the stethoscope at the apex. A III/VI, coarse crescendo-decrescendo murmur is heard at the upper right sternal border with radiation to the carotids. In addition, there is a II/VI early diastolic blowing murmur heard at the upper and mid-loft sternal border. The remainder of the examination is within normal limits.

ADDITIONAL DATA

The chest x-ray shows mild cardiomegaly and interstitial pulmonary edema. The ECG shows sinus tachycardia with a left anterior superior hemiblock. The white blood count is 13,600 mm3 with 83% segmented forms and 6% band forms. The hemoglobin 12.0 g/dl.

CLUE FROM THE HISTORY AND EXAMINATION

This patient presents with fever, a change in her systolic murmur, and the development of aortic regurgitation with mild to moderate congestive heart failure.

QUESTIONS

1. What is the most likely diagnosis and the most common etiologic agent(s)?
2. How should the diagnosis be established/confirmed?
3. What initial therapy should be instituted?

ANSWERS

1.  Infective endocarditis (IE) of the aortic valve. The most common cause of subacute bacterial endocarditis is streptococcus viridans, which may be responsible for over 50% of cases. Other relatively common organisms are: enteroccocus, group D (nonenterococcal) streptococcus, and staphylococcus epidermidis (especially with prosthetic valve endocarditis).
2.  The diagnosis of IE is based on the demonstration of multiple blood cultures positive for the responsible organism in the appropriate clinical setting. As the bacteremia associated with IE is thought to be continuous, only a relatively small number of blood cultures is required. Three sets of blood cultures (vented and unvented) should be obtained initially, and if the cultures are negative at 24 hours, 2 additional sets should be obtained the following day.
3.  Digitalis and furosemide should be instituted for the treatment of this patient's heart failure secondary to aortic regurgitation. In patients who are hemodynamically stable and who do not have "acute" endocarditis, it is safe to wait for 24-48 hours to institute antimicrobial therapy until culture results are available.

HOSPITAL COURSE

On the 2nd hospital day, 3 of 3 cultures are positive for a streptococcus viridans (nonenterococcus), and high-dose intravenous penicillin is begun. Over the next 3 days the patient develops increasing signs of aortic insufficiency and worsening of her congestive heart failure. In addition, she evidences new left bundle branch block (LBBB).

QUESTIONS

4.  How would you document the appropriateness of the antimicrobial regimen?
5.  What is the significance of the conduction abnormalities?
6.  What further therapy is indicated?

ANSWERS

4. The minimal bactericidal concentration (MBC) is the concentration of antimicrobial agent required to kill 99.9% of the original inoculum. The mean inhibitory concentration (MIC) is the lowest concentration needed to inhibit growth. An MIC of less than 0.1-0.2 mcg/ml for penicillin defines extremely sensitive strains of streptococci for which penicillin therapy alone is adequate. Serum killing levels (SKL) of 1:8 (the ability of the patient's serum to kill the organism at a dilution of 1:8 following the dose of antimicrobial) is used by some to confirm the adequacy of antimicrobial therapy.

5. Conduction system abnormalities, such as left bundle branch block (LBBB) in the setting of IE of the aortic valve, may be the first sign of extension of the infection to the valve ring and possible valve ring abscess.

6. This patient has both aortic insufficiency with congestive heart failure and new LBBB as complications of aortic valve endocarditis. These are 2 indications for surgical intervention, and thus cardiac catheterization should be done as a prelude to aortic valve replacement. Additional indications for valve surgery in IE include: uncontrolled infection, fungal endocarditis, recurrent systemic emboli, and mechanical complication such as rupture of a sinus of Valsalva or ventricular septal defect.

PEARLS

1. Organisms such as staphylococcus aureus, pneumococcus, neisseria species and hemophilus influenzae are more frequently associated with the "acute" form of infective endocarditis.

2. In proven bacterial endocarditis, the first 3 sets of cultures will be positive in 95% of patients who ultimately are "culture positive."

3. In streptococcus viridans endocarditis, the first culture will be positive in over 90% of cases.

4. There are 4 major embolic findings in subacute IE: petechaie, splinter (subungual) hemorrhages, Osler nodes (tender, erythematous, raised lesions of the pulps of the fingers and toes and on the palms) and Janeway lesions (nontender, flat lesions of the palms and soles).

5. Two-dimensional echocardiography is likely to demonstrate the valvular vegetations of IE in 80% of patients and may well show

suppurative complications of IE, such as abscess or purulent pericarditis.
6. A sudden hemiplegia or other CNS event in a young person should raise the possibility of endocarditis. Neurologic events may result from rupture of a mycotic aneurysm, embolization or meningeal infection.
7. The relapse rate following 4 weeks of high-dose intravenous penicillin therapy for penicillin-sensitive streptococcus viridans IE is approximately 1%.

## PITFALLS

1. Antimicrobial thorapy in the preceding 2 weeks may markedly decrease the yield of blood cultures in patients wlth IE.
2. Due to earlier diagnosis and treatment, Osler nodes and Janeway lesions are seen in fewer than 20% of patients with the subacute form of IE.
3. Cultures are negative in 10-15% of cases of IE; this may be due to recent antimicrobial therapy, improper culture techniques, special growth requirements of the organism, or the presence of fungal endocarditis. Routine subculturing of broth at 48 hours onto special media is recommended when fastidious organisms are suspected.
4. Valve thickening, calcification and other abnormalities of the valve leaflets may appear identical to vegetations of IE on 2-dimensional echocardiography.
5. Vegetations may persist indefinitely in patients with IE despite appropriate therapy; this is not indicative of failure of the antimicrobial therapy to eradicate the infection.

## REFERENCES

Martin RP, Meltzer RS, Chia BL, et al: Clinical utility of two dimensional echocardiography in infective endocarditis. Am J Cardiol 46:379, 1980.

McAnulty JH, Rahimtoola SH: Surgery for infective endocarditis. JAMA 242:77, 1979.

Reid CL, Chandraratna PAN, Rahimtoola SH: Infective endocarditis: Improved diagnosis and treatment. Curr Probl Cardiol 10:6, 1985.

Washington JA II: The role of the microbiology laboratory in the diagnosis and antimicrobial treatment of infective endocarditis. Mayo Clin Proc 57:22, 1982.

Wilson WR, Giuliani ER, Geraci JE:    Treatment of penicillin-sensitive
streptococcal infective endocarditis.   Mayo Clin Proc 57:95, 1982.

## CASE 12: DYSPNEA AND CHANGING HEART MURMUR

HISTORY

A 48-year-old woman with a history of a heart murmur complains of increasing fatigue and breathlessness over the past 2 weeks. In her 20's she was told that she had a click and a "mildly leaky" valve. She is on no medication except for antibiotics prior to dental procedures. She denies excessive salt intake, palpitations, chest pressure or fevers. There is no history of rheumatic fever.

EXAMINATION

On examination she is mildly short of breath at rest, with a regular heart rate of 96, a blood pressure of 120/76, and a temperature of 36.8ºC. The jugular pulsations are normal, and the venous pressure is estimated at 10 cm of water. The carotid pulse is tapping in quality with a sharp upstroke. There are rales 1/3 of the way up the chest. The left ventricular (LV) impulse is in the anterior axillary line in the 6th intercostal space. There is a left parasternal lift and an apical systolic thrill. The 1st heart sound is prominent with widened splitting of the 2nd heart sound. A grade IV/VI systolic murmur beginning shortly after S1 and lasting throughout systole is appreciated at the apex and into the axilla and can be heard with the stethoscope applied to the midcervical spine.

ADDITIONAL DATA

The ECG shows sinus rhythm with left atrial enlargement. The chest x-ray reveals mild cardiomegaly with a cardiothoracic ratio of 0.54. There is straightening of the left heart border below the pulmonary artery; vascular redistribution is present.

CLUE FROM THE HISTORY AND EXAMINATION

This patient with previously well-tolerated, chronic mitral regurgitation (MR) presents with a relatively sudden increase of her murmur, an acceleration of her symptoms, and congestive heart failure.

QUESTIONS

1. What is the most likely cause of this patient's underlying valvular disease?
2. What might be responsible for the exacerbation of her symptoms?
3. What initial diagnostic test(s) would you order?
4. What initial treatment is indicated?
5. Is cardiac catheterization necessary in this patient?
6. Should mitral valve surgery be performed in this patient?

ANSWERS

1.  Primary myxomatous degeneration of the mitral valve (the most common cause of mitral regurgitation) is the cause of this patient's regurgitation. Other common etiologies include ischemic heart disease and rheumatic heart disease.
2.  Rupture of one or more chordae tendineae is a common cause of acute worsening of mitral regurgitation in patients with myxomatous mitral valve disease. Other causes of decompensation include atrial fibrillation, endocarditis and excess salt intake.
3.  An echocardiogram would help differentiate between rheumatic mitral valve disease and myxomatous degeneration. More importantly, LV and left atrial dimensions can be measured and overall wall motion assessed. Doppler technique can confirm and estimate the degree of mitral regurgitation. Blood cultures should also be sent to exclude infective endocarditis.
4.  The patient's heart failure should be controlled with furosemide and digitalis. Vasodilator therapy may be required if initial therapy is not readily successful. One might consider hemodynamic monitoring with a Swan-Ganz catheter to assess the need for vasodilators and the response to therapy.
5.  The patient has developed moderate to severe heart failure, and it is unlikely that medical treatment alone will return her to normal exercise tolerance. Following stabilization, cardiac catheterization should be considered to quantify the degree of regurgitation, measure left- and right-sided pressures, and look for occult coronary artery disease or other unsuspected valvular abnormality.
6.  Patients with limiting symptoms and without severe LV dysfunction have improved functional status and survival following successful mitral valve replacement. Furthermore, mitral valve repair with plication of the mitral valve annulus without valve replacement may be feasible in some patients with myxomatous degeneration.

PEARLS

1.  Myxomatous degeneration of the mitral valve has supplanted rheumatic disease as the most common cause of mitral regurgitation requiring mitral valve replacement.
2.  Mitral regurgitation due to rheumatic heart disease is characteristically associated with a decrease in the intensity of S1

due to shortening of the subvalvular apparatus and decreased ability of the valve to close.

3. Murmurs of mitral regurgitation may radiate posteriorly and be transmitted to the spine and conducted by bone as high as the top of the skull.

4. Survival of patients undergoing mitral valve replacement for mitral regurgitation is dependent on the etiology of the valvular disease. Five-year survival following mitral valve replacement for myxomatous or rheumatic mitral disease is greater than 50%, as compared with 30% for mitral regurgitation due to ischemic heart disease. Preoperative functional class is another major factor that determines long-term survival after valve replacement.

5. There is no direct means by which the echocardiographic diagnosis of mitral regurgitation can be made; indirect evidence for MR includes left atrial enlargement, valvular abnormalities, and findings of LV volume overload.

PITFALLS

1. In severe mitral regurgitation, the ejection fraction, as measured by contrast or nuclear ventriculography, markedly underestimates the degree of impairment because the left ventricle empties into the low-pressure left atrium.

2. Chronic MR may be tolerated for years, if not decades, in many patients without apparent deterioration in LV function. Premature valve replacement would thus subject patients unnecessarily to years of anticoagulation and other risks of "prosthetic valve disease." However, patients with chronic MR may develop significant and irreversible LV dysfunction before they develop limiting symptoms. Unfortunately, it is not clear what the optimal time is for mitral valve replacement in asymptomatic patients to prevent irreversible LV dysfunction.

REFERENCES

DePace NL, Nestico PF, Morganroth J: Acute severe mitral regurgitation: Pathophysiology, clinical recognition and management. Am J Med 78:293, 1985.

Fleming HA, Bailey SM: Mitral valve disease, systemic embolism and anticoagulants. Postgrad Med J 47:599, 1971.

Hammermeister KE, Fisher L, Kennedy JW, et al: Prediction of late survival in patients with mitral valve disease from clinical, hemodynamic and quantitative angiographic variables. Circulation 57:341, 1978.

Rahimtoola SH: Valvular heart disease: A perspective. J Am Coll Cardiol 1:199, 1983.

## CASE 13: DIASTOLIC MURMUR IN A YOUNG MAN

HISTORY

A 28-year-old truck driver presents with symptoms of mild fatigue and dyspnea with extreme exertion.  A murmur detected during an army physical prevented him from enlisting in the armed services, and he vaguely recalls the mention of an "abnormality" during a routine examination prior to participating in high-school football.  He has no history of rheumatic fever, chest pain, orthopnea or edema.  Palpitations, described as a forceful impulse in the chest, have been noted, especially while lying on his left side or following activity.  He denies fever, rash, recent dental work, chest trauma, syncope or back pain.

EXAMINATION

Examination shows a tall, slender young man with no clubbing or cyanosis. Blood pressure is 140/40; heart rate is 85; respirations are 20.  The lung fields are clear.  There are prominent and bounding pulses throughout.  The carotid upstroke has a bisferiens contour.  The jugular venous pressure is 7 cm of $H_2O$.  The left ventricular impulse is 2 cm left of the midclavicular line and is hyperdynamic.  There is a normal 1st heart sound and an attenuated aortic component to the 2nd heart sound.  A grade III/VI systolic ejection murmur and a grade III/VI diastolic, high-pitched, decrescendo murmur, heard best at the left 3rd-5th intercostal spaces, are noted.  A diastolic bruit is heard over the femoral artery when the stethoscope is compressed against it.  The abdomen is benign, and the extremities show no edema.

ADDITIONAL DATA

The chest x-ray shows moderate cardiomegaly with normal pulmonary vascularity, a prominent aortic root and a large convex left ventricle extending below the left hemidiaphragm.

The ECG shows left axis deviation and left ventricular (LV) hypertrophy with strain.

An echocardiogram and Doppler flow study are shown below:

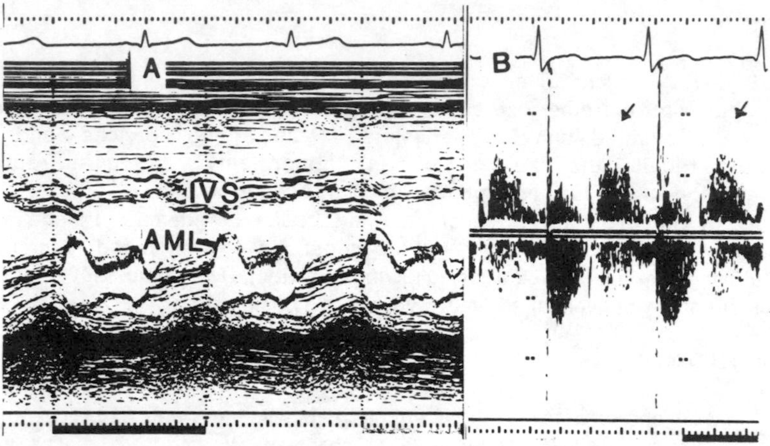

INTERPRETATION OF ECHOCARDIOGRAM AND DOPPLER:  Figure A is an M mode tracing at the level of the mitral valve and shows diastolic fluttering of the anterior mitral leaflet (AML).  IVS = interventricular septum.  Figure B is a pulsed-wave Doppler tracing with the transducer aimed along the long axis of the left ventricle from the cardiac apex.  The arrows point to regurgitant flow toward the transducer.

QUESTIONS

1.  What are the possible etiologies for aortic regurgitation in this young man?
2.  What are common physical findings in severe aortic regurgitation?
3.  What studies will help define the severity and etiology of the valvular lesion and provide a tool for follow-up and evaluation?
4.  What parameters of LV function are used to decide the timing of surgery?  What guidelines should be followed to select patients for aortic valve replacement?

ANSWERS

1.  The common causes of aortic regurgitation that might apply to this case include a congenital bicuspid aortic valve, rheumatic heart disease, myxomatous degeneration of the aortic valve, connective tissue diseases including Marfan's syndrome, and infective endocarditis. Less common etiologies include aortitis (e.g., syphilis or Takayasu's disease), aortic dissection and ankylosing spondylitis.

2.  Physical findings compatible with severe chronic regurgitation include a bisferiens contour of the carotid impulse and an increased pulse pressure. Auscultation shows an aortic systolic murmur, a long and high-pitched diastolic murmur and, occasionally, a diastolic rumbling murmur (Austin Flint). Quincke's capillary pulsations are notable on the nails; Duroziez's murmur with a diastolic sound over a partially compressed femoral artery, Corrigan's water-hammer pulses, and DeMusset's "head-bob" are additional findings.

3.  The echocardiogram will provide anatomical information about the etiology by showing details of valvular structure, aortic root size and LV wall thickness and should be a part of the early work-up. Systolic function may be defined by echocardiography or by radionuclide ventriculography, which are useful for follow-up and decision-making regarding the timing of valve surgery.

4.  The most common methods of following LV systolic function are the ejection fraction (radionuclide technique) and the percent fractional shortening and end-systolic dimension (echocardiography). No exact lower limits have been defined beyond which aortic valve replacement is contraindicated; however, the prognosis for recovery is poor, with severely depressed function (ejection fraction of 30% or less). Operative intervention is recommended for patients who have severe aortic regurgitation and marked symptoms (New York Heart Association class III or IV). Minimally symptomatic patients (class I or II) may be considered for surgery if there is evidence of progressive deterioration of left ventricular function.

PEARLS

1.  Chronic aortic regurgitation is often well tolerated for years, despite evidence of cardiac enlargement.

2.  Symptoms of angina, congestive heart failure and syncope (harbingers of a poor prognosis in aortic stenosis) likewise occur with severe

of a poor prognosis in aortic stenosis) likewise occur with severe aortic regurgitation.

3. The ejection sound typical of a bicuspid aortic valve is absent when regurgitation is severe, but it is present (usually at the apex) when incompetence is mild or moderate.

4. The etiologic factors in aortic regurgitation can be usefully separated into 2 groups: those affecting the aortic valve itself (e.g., rheumatic, congenital, endocarditis, myxomatous) and those affecting the aortic root (e.g., dissection, hypertension, Marfan's, aortitis, trauma).

PITFALLS

1. Insertion of an intra-aortic balloon pump is contraindicated in aortic regurgitation.

2. Symptoms of LV dysfunction may be subtle and develop quite gradually, underscoring the value of serial examinations and noninvasive assessment. The development of significant symptoms with aortic regurgitation, although less frequent than with aortic stenosis, may be followed by rapid deterioration.

3. Test variability in echo measurements is a problem. Dimensional changes varying 10% from baseline may only reflect variation in technique.

4. Sudden worsening of symptoms in a patient with "stable" aortic regurgitation may indicate the onset of infective endocarditis, myocardial infarction or significant dysrhythmias.

REFERENCES

Cheitlin MD:  The timing of surgery in mitral and aortic valve diseases. Circ Pub in Cardiology 12:69, 1987.

Fioretti P, Roelandt J, Bos RJ, et al:  Echocardiography in aortic insufficiency:  Is valve replacement too late when left ventricular end systolic dimension reaches 55 mm?  Circulation 67:216, 1983.

Fortuin NJ, Craige E:  On the mechanisms of the Austin Flint murmur. Circulation 45:558, 1972.

Greenberg BH:  Aortic insufficiency:  Vasodilator therapy.  Primary Cardiol 8:35, 1982.

Henry WL, Bonow RO, Borer JS, et al:  Observations on the optimum time

Perloff JK:   The Clinical Recognition of Congenital Heart Disease. Philadelphia, WB Saunders, 1987.

Segal J, Harvey WW, Hufnagle CA:   Clinical study of 100 cases of severe aortic insufficiency.   Am J Med 21:200, 1956.

Szlachcic J, Massie BM, Greenberg B, et al:   Intertest variability of echocardiographic and chest x-ray measurements:   Implications for decision making in patients with aortic regurgitation.   J Am Coll Cardiol 7:1310, 1986.

## CASE 14: LONG-STANDING HEART MURMUR AND PROGRESSIVE FATIGUE

HISTORY

A 55-year-old farmer presents with exertional fatigue, dyspnea, mild ankle edema and the recent onset of palpitations. He has noted a mild reduction in exercise tolerance over the past 8 months, and routine chores have been causing a rapid, irregular chest pounding. No dizziness or syncope has occurred. There is no history of rheumatic fever, recent dental work, fever or chills, and he denies chest pain. A murmur was detected 10 years ago, and 3 years ago a chest x-ray for a routine physical showed "borderline cardiomegaly."

EXAMINATION

The physical examination shows an alert, oriented, well-developed and well-nourished white male in no acute distress. There is no clubbing or cyanosis. Blood pressure is 110/70; heart rate is 130 and irregular. The neck is supple without thyromegaly, and the lungs are notable for right basilar rales. The cardiovascular exam shows a jugular venous pressure of 9 cm of $H_2O$, and the left ventricular (LV) impulse is felt 2 cm left of the midclavicular line in the 6th intercostal space. There is a 3rd heart sound. A grade III/VI holosystolic, harsh murmur is best heard at the LV apex. Radiation is noted primarily toward the axilla and heard faintly in the back along the spine. There is no diastolic murmur. The peripheral pulses are normal, and trace pedal edema is present.

ADDITIONAL DATA

The chest x-ray shows moderate cardiomegaly, mild redistribution of pulmonary blood flow and Kerley B lines. The ECG shows left ventricular hypertrophy; the rhythm strip is shown below:

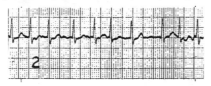

QUESTIONS

1.  What are the characteristic physical findings of mitral regurgitation (MR)?
2.  Why did decompensation occur in this setting?
3.  What are the most common etiologies of chronic mitral regurgitation?
4.  What are reasonable criteria for recommending cardiac catheterization?   Surgical intervention?

ANSWERS

1.  The mitral regurgitation murmur is holosystolic and is exacerbated by hand grip exercise, by squatting and by applying blood pressure cuffs to both upper extremities to cause transient arterial occlusion. The Valsalva maneuver, standing, and amyl nitrate inhalation reduce the intensity of the murmur. The regurgitant murmur radiates to the axilla but may also radiate to the base (mimicking aortic stenosis), in the case of rupture of posterior chordal attachment, or to the spine or even the top of the head, in the case of anterior leaflet rupture. S1 is often reduced, though it may be prominent in MR associated with mitral valve prolapse (MVP), and S2 is often widely split due to the shortening of LV ejection, resulting in an earlier A2.

2.  Hemodynamic decompensation occurred when atrial fibrillation developed. When the atrial contribution to LV filling is lost in the setting of chronic severe MR, cardiac output may decrease by 20-30%, resulting in a dramatic worsening of symptoms. Other causes of decompensation include rupture of chordal attachments, bacterial endocarditis and ischemic papillary muscle dysfunction.

3.  A competent mitral valve (MV) depends on the integrity of several components: leaflets, annulus, chordae tendineae and papillary muscles. Recent surgical pathology studies have shown that myxomatous degeneration (with mitral valve prolapse) is now more common than rheumatic disease in patients undergoing mitral valve replacement for regurgitation. Infection, trauma, ischemia and connective tissue disease also cause mitral regurgitation.

4.  Cardiac catheterization in MR is indicated whenever symptoms suggesting LV dysfunction develop or when progressive LV dysfunction is clearly demonstrated by noninvasive studies, even in the absence of symptoms. Symptoms usually indicate that a falloff in LV ejection fraction (LVEF) or an elevation of pulmonary pressure has occurred, and this may be demonstrated at the time of cardiac catheterization. Valve replacement is indicated for symptomatic, severe MR even if the LVEF is within normal limits. Surgery may also be recommended in asymptomatic patients with severe MR who show mild to moderate deterioration in left ventricular function.

PEARLS

1. The prognosis for chronic MR is quite variable, depending upon the etiology, with the presence of coronary artery disease being predictive of a poor long-term outcome, a rheumatic etiology providing an intermediate prognosis, and MVP with myxomatous degeneration being associated with the best long-term outlook.
2. Vasodilator therapy can provide a marked improvement in symptoms, since a reduction in afterload will result in improved forward flow and a reduction in pulmonary venous congestion. Hydralazine, captopril and enalapril are examples of such drugs.
3. Open valvuloplasty (surgical repair) is an alternative to mitral valve replacement in certain patients with prolapse and chordal rupture. Annular dilation can be reduced by insertion of a device such as the Carpentier ring.
4. Although MVP more commonly affects women, severe myxomatous MR requiring MV replacement is more common in men.

PITFALLS

1. Timing of MV replacement for chronic MR is one of the most difficult decisions in clinical cardiology.
2. The LV ejection fraction is an insensitive marker of LV dysfunction in MR, because the low-pressure left atrium effectively "afterload reduces" the left ventricle. This may explain why LVEF may fall after successful MV replacement.
3. Dysrhythmias other than atrial fibrillation are also common. Frequent premature ventricular complexes, atrial flutter and rare cases of ventricular tachycardia or fibrillation are noted with severe MR.

REFERENCES

Abbasi AS, Allen MV, DeCristofaro D, et al: Detection and estimation of the degree of mitral regurgitation by range-gated pulsed Doppler echocardiography. Circulation 61:143, 1980.
Lembo NJ, Dell Italia LJ, Crawford MH, O'Rourke RA: Diagnosis of left-sided regurgitant murmurs by transient arterial occlusion: A new maneuver using blood pressure cuffs. Ann Intern Med 105:368, 1986.
Pons-Llod G, Carreras-Cost F, Ballester-Rodes M, et al: Pulsed Doppler

patterns of left atrial flow in mitral regurgitation. Am J Cardiol 57: 806, 1986.

Tresch DD, Doyle TP, Borchek LI, et al: Mitral valve prolapse requiring surgery: Clinical and pathologic study. Am J Med 70:245, 1985.

Waller BF, Morrow AG, Morrow BJ, et al: Etiology of clinically isolated severe, chronic, pure mitral regurgitation: Analysis of 97 patients over 30 years of age having mitral valve replacement. Am Heart J 104:276,1982.

## CASE 15: EXERTIONAL ANGINA AND A HEART MURMUR

HISTORY

A 50-year-old football coach presents with dyspnea noticed while running in practice. For the past few months he has had exertional chest tightness and some slight dizziness. He was first told about a heart murmur during a routine grammar-school physical exam.

EXAMINATION

On examination, the patient has a blood pressure of 105/80 and a heart rate of 75. His carotid upstroke is delayed, but the amplitude of the pulse is normal. There is no right ventricular heave, and the prominent left ventricular impulse is in the 5th intercostal space in the midclavicular line. There is a regular rate and rhythm and a decreased aortic closure sound. A 4th heart sound is present. A III/VI late-peaking systolic ejection murmur is heard at the 2nd intercostal space along the right sternal border, radiating to the suprasternal notch. There is a II/VI holosystolic murmur along the left sternal border and the apex. No diastolic murmur is heard. The lungs are clear to auscultation. There is no peripheral edema.

ADDITIONAL DATA

The chest x-ray is reported as normal.

The ECG and echocardiogram with Doppler are shown below:

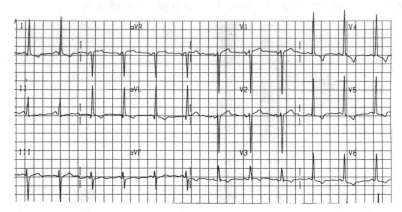

INTERPRETATION OF ECG:  Left ventricular hypertrophy with strain pattern.

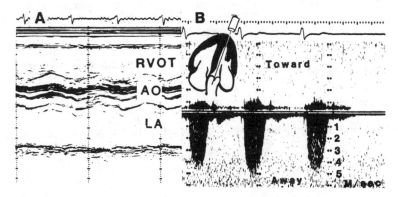

INTERPRETATION OF ECHO-DOPPLER:  Figure A is an M mode view through the aortic valve (AO) that shows thickened leaflets with reduced opening. LA = left atrium; RVOT = right ventricular outflow tract.  Figure B is a continuous wave Doppler recording with an apical transducer position demonstrating high-velocity flow (4-5 m/second) away from the transducer.

QUESTIONS

1. What is the most likely diagnosis?
2. What is the classic triad of symptoms in left ventricular (LV) outflow obstruction?
3. What are the physical findings which help differentiate this problem from hypertrophic cardiomyopathy?
4. What are the most common etiologies of this condition? Which is most likely in this patient?
5. What is the natural history of this problem?
6. What is the most appropriate work-up at this point in the patient's course?
7. What is the treatment?

ANSWERS

1. Valvular aortic stenosis.
2. The classic triad of symptoms in LV outflow obstruction are: angina, syncope and dyspnea.
3. The carotid upstroke is delayed (pulsus tardus) in aortic stenosis, as opposed to the rapid upstroke and bisferiens quality of the pulse in hypertrophic cardiomyopathy. The heart murmur increases in intensity with the Valsalva maneuver in hypertrophic cardiomyopathy and does not increase with aortic stenosis. A 4th heart sound is common to both problems.
4. The 3 most common etiologies of aortic stenosis in the adult are: congenital bicuspid aortic valve, rheumatic heart disease and degenerative calcific disease. The most likely etiology in this case is a congenital bicuspid aortic valve, which is more common in males and typically presents with symptoms in the 5th and 6th decades.
5. Symptoms often occur late in the course of the natural history of aortic stenosis. The occurrence of symptoms implies a poor prognosis with a 5-year mortality of greater than 50%.
6. Confirmation by cardiac catheterization is strongly indicated in this case. Determining the aortic valve area, as well as assessing the presence of any coexistent disease in other valves, is important. Although the left ventricle is hypertrophied, the LV contractility is usually well preserved until very late in the course when the left ventricle dilates. Coronary angiography is indicated at the time of catheterization.
7. Surgery with aortic valve replacement is considered when the aortic valve area is less than 1.0 cm2 (normal, 2.6-3.5 cm2).

PEARLS

1. Regardless of etiology, all cases of adult aortic stenosis are associated with calcification of the valve. This calcification can be readily seen on routine fluoroscopy, which is a simple way to confirm the diagnosis.
2. Angina pectoris is common in adult patients with aortic stenosis. In those patients with normal coronary arteries, angina is due to the ischemia produced by the increased demands of a thick, hypertrophic left ventricle. However, coexistent coronary artery disease must be

excluded at the time of heart catheterization.

3.  Echocardiography is a valuable diagnostic tool in evaluating the presence of cusp calcification, decreased mobility, other associated valvular abnormalities, chamber size and wall thickness. Doppler echocardiography can be used to estimate the peak gradient across the valve and gives some indication of the severity of the stenosis.

4.  Congestive heart failure is an ominous finding in aortic stenosis and is associated with 50% 2-year mortality. Despite the increased operative mortality with congestive heart failure, surgery still offers a substantial improvement over the natural history of the disease.

5.  Adults with critical aortic stenosis who are not operative candidates because of severe pulmonary or other diseases may be considered for palliation with balloon valvuloplasty.

PITFALLS

1.  The murmur of aortic stenosis, which is usually heard best at the upper sternal margins, is also often well heard across the precordium and the apex. The murmur becomes more holosystolic as it radiates to the apex, which is known as the Gallavardin phenomenon. It is often difficult to exclude the coexistence of mitral regurgitation.

2.  Older patients with atherosclerosis of the carotid vessels will often have what appears to be a normal carotid upstroke.

3.  Elderly patients with ejection murmurs may pose a diagnostic challenge. Aortic sclerosis is a common condition in the elderly; there is little or no obstruction to LV outflow, but there is an ejection murmur caused by fibrosis and calcification at the base of the cusps in the aortic root. The murmurs of aortic sclerosis may completely mimic that of aortic stenosis, and the differentiation may be extremely difficult, even for the experienced cardiologist. The sclerotic murmur is shorter, peaks earlier, and is associated with a normal aortic closure sound. The murmur of aortic stenosis is more prolonged, later peaking and often associated with a decreased aortic closure sound.

4.  Vasodilator drugs are potentially dangerous in aortic stenosis because of lowered blood pressure and decreased coronary blood flow.

5.  Exercise testing is dangerous and contraindicated in patients with severe aortic stenosis.

REFERENCES

Cribier A, Savin T, Berland J, et al:   Percutaneous transluminal balloon valvuloplasty of adult aortic stenosis:   Report of 92 cases.   J Am Coll Cardiol 9:381, 1987.

Frank S, Johnson A, Ross J Jr.:   Natural history of valvular aortic stenosis. Br Heart J 35:41, 1973.

Johnson AD, Engler RL, LeWinter M, et al:   The medical and surgical management of patients with aortic valve disease:   A symposium. West J Med 126:460, 1977.

Rahimtoola SH:   Outcome of aortic valve surgery.   Circulation 60:1191, 1979.

Selzer A:   Changing aspects of the natural history of valvular aortic stenosis.   N Engl J Med 317:91, 1987.

## CASE 16: PALPITATIONS AND HEART FAILURE IN A MIDDLE-AGED WOMAN

HISTORY

A 48-year-old Hispanic woman presents with rapid palpitations, fatigue and dyspnea with mild exertion. She has never been to a doctor and has no previous history of cardiovascular symptoms except some increasing tiredness over the past year. She is the mother of 7 children and works at her home as a seamstress. She denies any unusual past illnesses but did have childhood infections with measles and chickenpox.

EXAMINATION

Physical examination reveals a well-developed, well-nourished female with a blood pressure of 105/70, an irregular pulse of 140, and a respiratory rate of 18. S1 is loud, S2 is normal, and there is no S3 or S4. There is a weak tapping left ventricular impulse and a faint RV lift along the left sternal border. An opening snap is heard shortly after S2, and a presystolic murmur is heard. Her lungs are clear to auscultation and percussion. The rest of her examination is within normal limits.

ADDITIONAL DATA

A chest x-ray shows straightening of the left upper heart border and elevation of the left main-stem bronchus.

The rhythm strip prior to treatment is shown below:

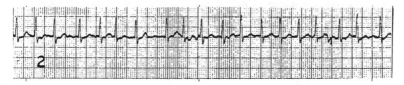

The ECG after initial treatment is shown below:

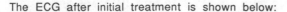
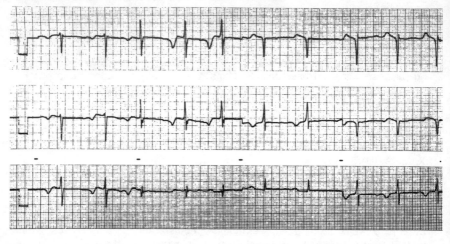

INTERPRETATION OF RHYTHM STRIP AND ECG: Atrial fibrillation with a controlled ventricular response rate; right ventricular hypertrophy; nonspecific ST-T wave changes.

QUESTIONS

1. What is the most likely diagnosis, based on the physical findings?
2. What is the rhythm on the ECG? What role does the arrhythmia play in the clinical presentation?
3. What noninvasive test will confirm the diagnosis? Can the severity of the lesion be assessed?
4. What is the medical treatment?
5. When is surgery recommended?

ANSWERS

1.  Mitral stenosis is the most likely diagnosis, based on the loud S1, the opening snap and the presystolic murmur.
2.  Atrial fibrillation with a rapid ventricular response rate is present on the rhythm strip. This plays an important role, in that the tachycardia causes a decrease in diastolic filling time and will often precipitate a clinical deterioration. Withdrawal of atrial contraction (as in atrial fibrillation) decreases cardiac output by approximately 20%.
3.  M mode echocardiography shows a thickened mitral valve, reduced EF slope, and diastolic anterior motion of the posterior leaflet. The valve area can be measured directly on the 2-dimensional study. Continuous wave Doppler shows the high flow through the mitral valve during a diastole, and a mitral valve gradient can be estimated. Using the clinical data, the echocardiogram and the Doppler study, the clinician can noninvasively assess the severity of the stenosis with a high degree of accuracy and good correlation with cardiac catheterization data.
4.  Control of the heart rate response is the most important initial therapy. This can be done with digitalis or propranolol to allow adequate diastolic filling time. Anticoagulation is indicated for this patient with atrial fibrillation and with a large left atrium. Bacterial endocarditis prophylaxis should be prescribed.
5.  Surgery is recommended for the Class III or IV patient whose calculated mitral valve area is less than 1 cm2 (normal, 4-5 cm2). Younger patients without marked calcification may benefit from mitral commissurotomy. Valve replacement is necessary if the valve is heavily calcified and immobile. Balloon valvulotomy offers a nonsurgical approach to increasing the valve area. This promising intervention is being studied extensively and may prove to be the treatment of choice for a substantial number of patients.

PEARLS

1.  Young patients with severe rheumatic disease may complain of fatigue and symptoms of right heart failure. "Protective" pulmonary hypertension is caused by pulmonary vasoconstriction, which keeps cardiac output low.
2.  Penicillin prophylaxis to prevent a recurrence of rheumatic fever is

indicated, particularly in patients exposed to high-population-density living or working environments.
3. Exercise testing may be an important tool in assessing the patient's functional capacity and in making decisions regarding the need for surgery.

PITFALLS

1. Acutely ill patients with pure mitral stenosis and congestive heart failure will generally further decompensate with rapid heart rates. Intravenous propranolol is the drug of choice to control the rate but is often withheld by the physician due to fear of aggravating the heart failure. This is an unwarranted concern in isolated mitral stenosis, as the left ventricle is normal.
2. Medical or electrical cardioversion should be approached with great caution or avoided in patients with atrial fibrillation and mitral stenosis. The enlarged left atrium leads to stagnation of blood and thrombus formation, which creates an increased risk of systemic embolization. Anticoagulation is necessary and appears to lower the risk of embolization.
3. A left atrial myxoma can simulate mitral stenosis, as both may present with clinical symptoms of pulmonary congestion. The pedunculated tumor may have a ball-valve effect, causing mitral obstruction as the tumor moves from the left atrium to the left ventricle. A loud 1st heart sound is common to both entities; an early diastolic thud ("tumor plop") can mimic an opening snap. Diastolic murmurs are heard in both.
4. Many patients with rheumatic valvular disease will not give a history of rheumatic fever.

REFERENCES

Kloster FG, Morris CD:  Natural history of valvular heart disease. Circulation 65:1283, 1982.
Rapaport E:  Natural history of aortic and mitral disease.  Am J Cardiol 35:221, 1975.
Roberts WC, Perloff JK:  Mitral valvular disease:  A clinicopathologic survey of the conditions causing the mitral valve to function abnormally.  Ann Intern Med 77:939, 1972.

## CASE 17: YOUNG WOMAN WITH CHEST PAINS AND PALPITATIONS

HISTORY

A 32-year-old female artist with intermittent sharp chest pains and heart pounding is referred for evaluation. Over the past few years she has had episodes of pain lasting several minutes to an hour, often associated with skipped beats. These episodes are most pronounced during times of stress. She is otherwise healthy and jogs up to 3 miles daily.

EXAMINATION

The patient is a tall, thin and anxious young woman in no distress. Heart rate is 84 and regular; blood pressure is 120/72. The jugular venous pulsations and the carotid upstroke are normal. There is a midsystolic, high-pitched sound at the lower sternal border, followed by a II/VI apical murmur that increases toward the end of systole.

ADDITIONAL DATA

The ECG shows nonspecific ST changes and unifocal premature ventricular contractions..

CLUE FROM THE M MODE ECHOCARDIOGRAM AND PHONOCARDIOGRAM

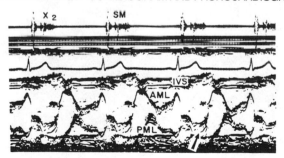

INTERPRETATION OF ECHOCARDIOGRAM AND PHONOCARDIOGRAM: The anterior mitral leaflet (AML) meets the elongated posterior mitral leaflet (PML) in middiastole. Shortly after normal systolic apposition of the leaflets, posterior bowing of both leaflets is seen (arrow). The nadir of this posterior movement coincides with 2 midsystolic clicks (X) and the beginning of a late systolic murmur (SM).

QUESTIONS

1. What is the diagnosis?
2. What symptoms are most common in this syndrome?
3. What maneuvers of bedside examination will help confirm the diagnosis?
4. What rhythm accounts for her "skipped beats"?
5. What is this patient's prognosis?
6. If this patient develops frequent and bothersome symptoms, what medication(s) would you recommend?

ANSWERS

1. Mitral valve prolapse (MVP), also called the click-murmur syndrome or Barlow's syndrome, is associated with myxomatous degeneration due to an unexplained abnormality of valvular collagen.
2. The most common symptoms are chest pain (often atypical for angina), palpitations, fatigue and syncope.
3. In mitral prolapse patients, the mitral valve is too big for the left ventricle, and this "valvulo-ventricular disproportion" can be made more prominent by certain maneuvers. The Valsalva maneuver, standing after squatting, and amyl nitrate inhalation all tend to decrease left ventricular volume and increase the disproportion between the chamber size and the relatively large mitral valve: the click moves closer to S1, and the murmur is accentuated.
4. Premature ventricular contractions (PVC's) are often perceived as skipped beats and are common in patients with MVP.
5. This patient should be reassured that the majority of patients with MVP have an excellent prognosis.
6. Beta-blocking agents are the most commonly used drugs in the treatment of symptomatic patients with MVP. These drugs are most helpful in those patients with adrenergic symptoms, such as heart pounding and tachyarrhythmias, and are less reliable in treating chest pain.

PEARLS

1. MVP is predominantly seen in women (with an incidence 10-20% of the female population).
2. MVP is seen in 10-20% of patients with secundum atrial septal defects. There is an increased association of MVP with other congenital heart problems, including anomalous bypass tracts, Marfan's syndrome, Ebstein's anomaly, and transposition of the great vessels.
3. Certain physical findings, such as thoracic cage abnormalities (kyphosis, pectus excavatum, straight back syndrome, scoliosis), joint hypermobility and tall stature, are seen with increased frequency in MVP patients.
4. The most common ECG abnormalities in MVP patients are nonspecific ST-T changes and premature beats.
5. Multiple valve prolapse (including tricuspid and aortic) is seen with

increased frequency in patients with Marfan's syndrome, Ehlers-Danlos syndrome and other systemic abnormalities of connective tissue.

## PITFALLS

1. Up to 20% of patients with a click and/or a murmur suggestive of MVP have false negative echocardiograms, even if 2-dimensional echocardiography is used. The physical examination remains the gold standard in the MVP syndrome.
2. Rare complications of MVP include embolic stroke, sudden cardiac death and endocarditis.
3. Patients with MVP and mitral regurgitation do have a small risk of bacterial endocarditis, and antibiotic prophylaxis for dental and other procedures associated with bacteremia is recommended by the American Heart Association. (Antibiotic prophylaxis for patients with clicks and no mitral regurgitation is controversial.)
4. A small percentage of patients with MVP, particularly those with both a click and a significant murmur, will develop progressive mitral insufficiency and ultimately require mitral valve surgery.

## REFERENCES

Barnett HJM, Boughner DR, Taylor DW, et al:  Further evidence relating mitral valve prolapse to cerebral ischemic events.  N Engl J Med 302:139, 1980.

Criley JM, Heger JW:  Prolapsed mitral leaflet syndrome.  In Roberts WC (ed):  Congenital Heart Disease in Adults.  Philadelphia, FA Davis, 1979.

Mills P,  Rose J, Hollingsworth J, et al:  Long-term prognosis of mitral valve prolapse.  N Engl J Med 297:13, 1977.

## CASE 18: SUDDEN DECOMPENSATION IN A MAN WITH A PROSTHETIC HEART VALVE

HISTORY

A 34-year-old sales manager is brought into the emergency room with 2 hours of severe substernal chest pressure and shortness of breath. He underwent mitral valve replacement with a Bjork-Shiley tilting disk prosthesis 3 years ago because of acute mitral regurgitation complicating infective endocarditis. According to his girlfriend, recently he has been feeling well, without dyspnea, chest pain, cough, fever or chills. However, he has been depressed since losing his job and has been taking his warfarin irregularly over the past few months.

EXAMINATION

Markedly dyspneic middle-aged man. Heart rate is 128 and regular; blood pressure is 84/64; respiration is 32. There is marked jugular venous distension, and the carotid pulse is decreased. Auscultation of the lungs reveals diffuse rales and wheezing. The opening click of the prosthetic valve is absent, and the closing sound is muffled. There is a summation gallop heard at the lower left sternal border but no systolic or diastolic murmur. Extremities are cold, and the peripheral pulses are diminished.

CLUE FROM THE HISTORY AND EXAMINATION

This man with a tilting disk prosthesis in the mitral position presents with acute pulmonary edema and diminished valve sounds. This is indicative of acute mechanical failure of the prosthesis.

QUESTIONS

1. What is the mechanism of this patient's valve failure?
2. What is the single most important risk factor for thrombosis of a mechanical valve?
3. What are other causes of mechanical failure of the prosthesis?
4. What noninvasive tests may help to confirm the diagnosis?
5. Should the patient undergo emergency cardiac catheterization?
6. What therapy is indicated?

ANSWERS

1. Acute failure of the tilting disk prosthesis is most likely due to thrombosis of the valve with obstruction.
2. Mechanical valve thrombosis usually occurs in the setting of inadequate systemic anticoagulation.
3. Acute valvular regurgitation may occur with the Bjork-Shiley valve, because of strut fracture with embolization of the disk. Paravalvular leak may be associated with any type of prosthetic valve. Infective endocarditis can result in prosthetic valvular dysfunction.
4. Echocardiography can show decreased disk motion and can occasionally identify valvular thrombus or vegetation; Doppler shows increased velocity of mitral inflow and a decreased effective valve area. A radio-opaque marker in the occluding disk of the valve allows for fluoroscopic assessment of disk motion.
5. When there is strong clinical evidence of acute prosthetic valve obstruction in a patient with severe hemodynamic compromise, cardiac catheterization presents an unnecessary risk and is not recommended.
6. Surgical exploration with valve debridement or replacement should be undertaken as soon as possible. Fibrinolytic therapy with intravenous streptokinase has been used in some patients with acute thrombosis of prosthetic valves who were felt to be at exceptionally high risk for surgical intervention.

PEARLS

1. Prosthetic valves in the mitral position, especially with small valve sizes or in the presence of left atrial enlargement or atrial fibrillation, have the highest risk of thrombotic occlusion which may exceed 10% incidence at 4 years.
2. Prosthetic valves present the greatest risk of infective endocarditis following procedures associated with bacteremia (e.g., dental work); intravenous antibiotic prophylaxis prior to such procedures is often used.
3. Infective endocarditis should be suspected, and blood cultures obtained, in any patient with a prosthetic heart valve who shows any change in cardiac status or valve function.
4. The addition of the antiplatelet agent dipyridamole to warfarin

anticoagulation decreases the risk of thromboembolic complications without significantly increasing the incidence of hemorrhage.
5. Thrombosis of the tilting disk prosthesis tends to occur suddenly and with higher mortality than thrombosis of the ball-in-cage prosthesis, which may be associated with symptoms of 1-3 months duration.

## PITFALLS

1. Although fibrinolytic therapy with intravenous streptokinase may be efficacious in acute prosthetic valve thrombosis, there is a significant risk of systemic embolization, and this mode of therapy should be considered only when emergency surgery is not feasible.
2. Fracture of the outlet strut causes catastrophic valve failure and has recently been recognized with the larger-size Bjork-Shiley valves in the mitral position.

## REFERENCES

Copans H, Lakier JB, Kinsley RH, et al: Thrombosed Bjork-Shiley mitral prostheses. Circulation 61:169, 1980.

Gore JM, Dalen JE: Complications of prosthetic heart valves: When to reoperate. J Cardiovasc Med (November):1153, 1983.

Kloster FE: Complications of artificial heart valves. JAMA 241:2201, 1979.

Kontos GJ Jr, Schaff HV: Thrombotic occlusion of a prosthetic heart valve: Diagnosis and management. Mayo Clin Proc 60:118, 1985.

Ledain LD, Ohayon JP, Colle JP, et al: Acute thrombotic obstruction with disc valve prosthesis: Diagnostic considerations and fibrinolytic treatment. J Am Coll Cardiol 7:743, 1986.

Wright JO, Hiratzka LF, Brandt B III, et al: Thrombosis of the Bjork-Shiley prosthesis: Illustrative cases and review of the literature. J Thorac Cardiovasc Surg 84:138,1982.

## CASE 19:  EXERTIONAL SYNCOPE IN AN ACTIVE YOUNG MAN

HISTORY

A 30-year-old basketball coach presents with a syncopal episode at the end of a long practice. He experienced some prolonged, sharp chest pain earlier in the day. He has no history of cold sweats, dyspnea or nausea. The patient has always been physically healthy and active with no history of smoking, hypertension or diabetes. His family history is significant in that his father died suddenly of an unknown cause at age 45.

EXAMINATION

Physical examination reveals a healthy, well-developed, Caucasian male in no acute distress. Vital signs are a blood pressure of 120/70, pulse of 65 and respirations of 14/minute. The jugular venous pulse shows a prominent A wave. The carotid pulse has a sharp, rapid rise and a bisferiens contour. His cardiac exam reveals an easily palpable left ventricular impulse in the 5th intercostal space at the midclavicular line with a palpable 4th sound. The 1st and 2nd heart sounds are normal, and there is a loud S4. A grade III/VI crescendo-decrescendo murmur is heard over the entire precordium and is also heard at the base and the axilla. After a Valsalva maneuver the murmur is markedly increased. There is no click. The rest of his exam is normal.

ADDITIONAL DATA

Initial studies produce normal laboratory test results, including normal cardiac enzymes and a normal cholesterol. A chest x-ray is also normal.

The patient's ECG is shown below:

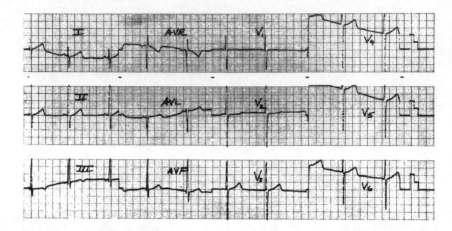

INTERPRETATION OF ECG: This tracing is recorded at 1/2 standard voltage. There is right axis deviation and evidence of right and left ventricular hypertrophy.

QUESTIONS

1. What is the diagnosis?
2. What test should be obtained to confirm the diagnosis?
3. What effect will dynamic maneuvers, such as the Valsalva, standing after squatting, and inhalation of amyl nitrate have on the murmur? (Explain the pathophysiology.)
4. Is cardiac catheterization necessary in this case?
5. What type of therapy would you recommend for this problem?

ANSWERS

1.  Hypertrophic cardiomyopathy (HCM). This disorder has also been called hypertrophic obstructive cardiomyopathy (HOCM), idiopathic hypertrophic subaortic stenosis (IHSS) and muscular subaortic stenosis (MSS).
2.  Echocardiography is usually diagnostic in this disease and is an invaluable tool. The typical features include asymmetric septal hypertrophy (septum-to-posterior wall thickness ratio of greater than 1.3), systolic anterior motion (SAM) of the anterior mitral valve leaflet, decreased EF slope, a normal or reduced left ventricular dimension and midsystolic closure of the aortic valve. This patient's M mode echocardiogram at the level of the mitral valve is shown below:

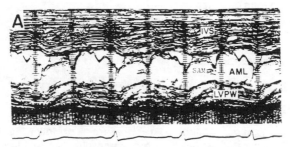

Figure A. AML = anterior mitral leaflet;
IVS = interventricular septum; LVPW =
left ventricular posterior wall

3.  The systolic murmur of HCM responds in a dynamic fashion to changes in preload (left ventricular volume), left ventricular contractility and left ventricular afterload. Valsalva, standing after squatting, and inhaling amyl nitrate all decrease left ventricular volume. With this decrease in cavity dimension, the anterior mitral leaflet and the interventricular system are brought dynamically closer into apposition, thus increasing the intensity of the murmur.
4.  Most cases of HCM can be diagnosed and managed effectively without cardiac catheterization. Certain situations may indicate the need for

invasive work-up, such as: (1) when the patient's chest pain and clinical profile are typical of angina and it may be necessary to ascertain the coronary anatomy, (2) when the noninvasive data are unclear, and (3) when the patient is being considered for cardiac surgery.

5.  Beta-adrenergic blockade is the mainstay of therapy and is most useful in alleviating chest pain.  It may be beneficial from an antiarrhythmic standpoint as well.  Doses in excess of 320 mg of propranolol per day are commonly used in the clinical management of these patients.  Calcium blockers, particularly verapamil, have been used because they decrease the forcefulness of contraction and may improve diastolic properties of the left ventricle.

## PEARLS

1.  Hypertrophic cardiomyopathy is found in many young athletes who die suddenly during or after exercise.
2.  Atrial arrhythmias are poorly tolerated by patients with HCM.  These should be treated aggressively.
3.  HCM may be familial (the majority have autosomal dominant transmission) or sporadic.

## PITFALLS

1.  A systolic pressure gradient may be present between the body of the left ventricle and the outflow tract, at rest or following provocation. Although this is considered by some to be evidence of an "obstruction," the variability of the gradient and the fact that the left ventricle ejects nearly its entire volume during the first half of systole suggests that there is no true impediment to flow.
2.  The significance of a pressure gradient is unclear.  There is a higher death rate in symptomatic patients with no gradient than those with a gradient.
3.  The clinical course of HCM is highly variable, and it is unclear how therapy alters the natural history.

REFERENCES

Criley JM, Lennon PA, Abbasi AS, et al:  Hypertrophic cardiomyopathy.  In Levine HJ (ed):  Clinical Cardiovascular Physiology.  New York, Grune and Stratton, 1976, pp 771-827.

Criley JM, Siegel RJ:  Has "obstruction" hindered our understanding of hypertrophic cardiomyopathy?  Circulation 72:1148, 1985.

Frank MJ, Abdulla M, Canedo MI, et al:  Long-term medical management of hypertrophic cardiomyopathy.  Am J Cardiol 42:993, 1978.

## CASE 20: YOUNG MAN WITH EDEMA, ABDOMINAL PAIN AND CARDIOMEGALY

HISTORY

A 27-year-old man comes to the office with 10 days of abdominal discomfort and swelling of his legs. The pain is dull and aching and is located in the right upper abdomen. Despite a decrease in his appetite, he has gained nearly 15 pounds. Four weeks ago he had a 2-week illness with a sore throat, fever and muscle aches. The past 2 nights he has awakened unable to catch his breath. Prior to the past 4 weeks, he has been healthy and active in sports without any limitations. He drinks alcohol infrequently. There is no history of heart disease or murmur and no family history of heart problems.

EXAMINATION

Heart rate is 110 with occasional premature beats; blood pressure is 100/76; respiration rate is 24. The jugular venous pressure is estimated at 14 cm of $H_2O$. The carotid pulse is decreased, and there are rales 1/3-1/2 of the way up the chest bilaterally. The left ventricular (LV) impulse is in the 7th intercostal space in the anterior axillary line; a left parasternal lift is present. There is a prominent 3rd heart sound and a III/VI holosystolic murmur at the apex, radiating to the axilla. The liver is tender and has a span of 15 cm to percussion. There is 3+ pitting edema to the knees.

ADDITIONAL DATA

The chest radiograph shows generalized cardiomegaly, pulmonary congestion and bilateral pleural effusions. The ECG reveals sinus tachycardia with left bundle branch block and frequent premature ventricular contractions.

QUESTIONS

1.  What is the cause of this patient's abdominal pain?
2.  What is his cardiac condition?
3.  What is his echocardiogram likely to show?
4.  What is the role of endomyocardial biopsy in this situation?
5.  What is this patient's prognosis?

ANSWERS

1. Right upper quadrant pain in the setting of acute right heart failure is likely due to liver congestion with stretching of the liver capsule.
2. Dilated cardiomyopathy (CM) is a primary heart muscle disorder not due to hypertensive, coronary artery, valvular, pericardial or congenital heart disease.
3. The echocardiogram will show enlargement and hypokinesis of both ventricles with little increase in wall thickness. The echocardiogram is useful to exclude primary valvular or pericardial causes and may show complications of dilated CM such as mural thrombus, pericardial effusion or secondary atrioventricular valve regurgitation by Doppler technique.

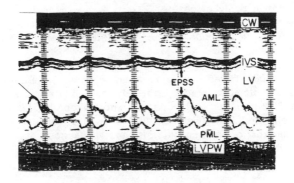

INTERPRETATION OF ECHOCARDIOGRAM: This shows both right ventricular (RV) and left ventricular (LV) enlargement and poor wall motion. The E point septal separation (EPSS) is markedly increased. AML = anterior mitral leaflet; CW = chest wall; IVS = interventricular septum; LVPW = left ventricular posterior wall; PML = posterior mitral leaflet.

4. Right ventricular endomyocardial biopsy via the transvenous approach may be useful in this setting of recent-onset dilated CM. The presence of lymphocytic infiltrates with ongoing muscle necrosis (i.e., myocarditis) may lead to the consideration of immuno-suppressive therapy with glucocorticosteroids and azothiaprine.

5. Dilated CM represents a heterogeneous group of diseases; however, the overall prognosis in a patient with severe heart failure is poor, and the average survival is less than 2 years.

## PEARLS

1. Patients with dilated cardiomyopathy may present with symptoms of systemic arterial embolization, such as a cerebral, mesenteric or renal infarction or a cold, pulseless extremity.
2. The murmur of mitral regurgitation in this patient is most likely due to displacement of the papillary muscles with failure of leaflet coaptation and is not due to primary valvular heart disease.
3. Although chamber dilatation is the main finding in dilated cardiomyopathy, there is an increase in LV wall thickness and muscle mass in the majority of cases.
4. Sudden cardiac death, presumably due to ventricular tachycardia or fibrillation, is a common cause of death in patients with dilated cardiomyopathy.
5. Recent trials have suggested that beta-blocking drugs in patients with idiopathic dilated cardiomyopathy are well tolerated and may improve symptomatic status and, possibly, short-term survival.
6. Biopsies in patients with dilated cardiomyopathy show myofibril hypertrophy and interstitial fibrosis, which are nonspecific findings. The hallmark of myocarditis is the presence of 5 or more lymphocytes/high-power field.

## PITFALLS

1. Although complex ventricular arrhythmias (e.g., multifocal or repetitive forms) are common in the cardiomyopathies, there is little proof that therapy of asymptomatic ventricular arrhythmias has any effect on long-term survival.
2. The use of immunosuppressive agents, even in patients with biopsy-proven myocarditis, is controversial and may be associated with potentially life-threatening complications.
3. The clinical diagnosis of myocarditis is unreliable, and as few as 10-25% of patients referred with this diagnosis will have evidence of lymphocytic myocarditis on biopsy.

REFERENCES

Dec GW Jr, Palacios IF, Fallon JT, et al: Active myocarditis in the spectrum of acute dilated cardiomyopathies. N Engl J Med 312:885, 1985.

Edwards WD: Myocarditis and endomyocardial biopsy. Cardiol Clin 2:647, 1984.

Engelmeier RS, O'Connell JB, Walsh R, et al: Improvement in symptoms and exercise tolerance by metoprolol in patients with dilated cardiomyopathy: A double-blind, randomized, placebo-controlled trial. Circulation 72:536, 1985.

Fowles RE, Mason JW: Role of cardiac biopsy in the diagnosis and management of cardiac disease. Prog Cardiovasc Dis 27:153, 1984.

Fuster V, Gersh BJ, Giuliani ER, et al: The natural history of idiopathic dilated cardiomyopathy. Am J Cardiol 47:525, 1981.

O'Connell JB, Henkin RE, Robinson JA, et al: Gallium-67 imaging in patients with dilated cardiomyopathy and biopsy-proven myocarditis.

## CASE 21: ENLARGED HEART IN A YOUNG NURSE

HISTORY

A 31-year-old nurse is found to have an enlarged heart on a routine chest x-ray. She has had "an innocent heart murmur" since birth but denies limitations in her activity or symptoms such as dyspnea, chest pain or palpitations. She reports frequent upper respiratory infections.

EXAMINATION

She is a slender, tall young woman. Heart rate is 82 and regular; blood pressure is 110/72 for right and left arms. Carotid upstroke and volume are normal, and jugular venous pressure is 5 cm H2O. The lungs are clear to auscultation without rales. There is a parasternal lift and a normal-sized left ventricular (LV) impulse in the 5th intercostal space in the midclavicular line. No thrill is present. Widened splitting of the 2nd heart sound is appreciated with little respiratory change. There is a II/VI crescendo-decrescendo murmur along the left sternal border, radiating to the suprasternal notch. Clubbing and cyanosis are absent.

ADDITIONAL DATA

The chest x-ray shows mild cardiomegaly with a cardiothoracic ratio of 0.55, right atrial and right ventricular prominence, and enlarged main pulmonary arteries with an increase in flow to the peripheral lung fields.

CLUE FROM THE ECG

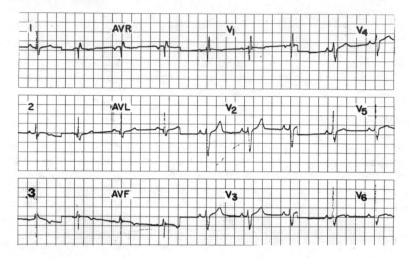

INTERPRETATION OF ECG: There is an rsR′ pattern in V1.

QUESTIONS

1. What is the functional/physiologic abnormality accounting for the abnormal chest x-ray and physical findings?
2. What specific cause of left-to-right shunt is suggested by the ECG in this young woman?
3. What complications occur in adults with this disorder?
4. When should surgical repair be recommended?

ANSWERS

1. The chest x-ray in this patient shows increased vascularity in the peripheral lung fields indicative of increased pulmonary arterial flow, which is the hallmark of a left-to-right intracardiac shunt.
2. The rsR´ configuration in V1 of the ECG with normal or right axis deviation is characteristic of an atrial septal defect of the secundum type (the most common type of ASD); ostium primum ASD is suggested by left and superior axis with the rsR´ in lead V1.
3. Complications of ASD in the adult include irreversible pulmonary hypertension and atrial tachyarrhythmias (e.g., atrial fibrillation) that may precipitato heart failure. The development of left-sided disease (such as coronary artery or hypertensive disease) decreases left ventricular compliance and thus increases the magnitude of the left-to-right shunt.
4. Surgical repair of an ASD is a very low-risk procedure in uncomplicated cases and is recommended when the ratio of pulmonary to systemic flow (Qp/Qs) exceeds 1.8-2.0 to 1. The majority of patients with clinically detectable ASD's have this degree of shunting. Qp/Qs may be accurately estimated by radionuclide techniques.

PEARLS

1. Fixed splitting of the 2nd heart sound in association with a pulmonic flow murmur is highly suggestive of ASD.
2. ASD's are often associated with gracile body habitus.
3. Up to 1/3 of patients with secundum ASD's have mitral valve prolapse.
4. The magnitude of the intracardiac shunt depends on the relative compliance of the left and right ventricles; normally, the highly compliant right ventricle results in predominantly left-to-right shunting.
5. ASD's of the sinus venous type (high in the atrial septum) are commonly associated with anomalous pulmonary veins that empty into the right atrium.
6. Infective endocarditis is rare in uncomplicated secundum ASD's; antibiotic prophylaxis is not generally recommended.

PITFALLS

1. Persistence of the splitting of the 2nd heart sound may occur in normal children or young adults; however, if normal, this should disappear with the patient sitting or standing.
2. Approximately 10-20% of adults with ASD will develop pulmonary hypertension and predominantly right-to-left shunting (Eisenmenger's physiology) which is irreversible and precludes surgical closure of the ASD.
3. Although ventricular septal defects are the most common cause of congenital left-to-right shunting, many close spontaneously, while others require surgical repair in childhood; atrial septal defects are thus the most common type of intracardiac shunt diagnosed in adults.
4. The development of atrial dysrrhythmias occurs in 25% of adults over the age of 45 with ASD and may cause dramatic worsening of their symptomatology.

REFERENCES

Fisher J, Platia EV, Weiss JL, Brinker JA: Atrial septal defect in the adult: Clinical findings before and after surgery. Cardiovasc Rev Rep 4:396, 1983.
Forfang K, Simonsen S, Anderson A, Efskind L: Atrial septal defect of secundum type in the middle aged. Am Heart J 94:44, 1977.
Heger JW, Niemann JT, Criley JM: Cardiology for the House Officer. Baltimore, Williams and Wilkins, 1987, pp 215-217.
Scully RE, Friedlich AL: Case records of the Massachusetts General Hospital: Case 13-1977. N Engl J Med 296:740, 1977.

## CASE 22: YOUNG WOMAN WITH CYANOSIS

HISTORY

A 21-year-old college female presents with symptoms of severe headache, dizziness and exertional chest pain. She has had a murmur since early childhood and has always been small for her age. For many years she has been unable to engage in physical education classes. Exertion has resulted in a dusky appearance and severe dyspnea accompanied by palpitations. These spells improve with lying down or squatting. She has a history of headaches, dizziness and nosebleeds.

EXAMINATION

Blood pressure is 98/60; heart rate is 96; respirations are 22. There is cyanosis and clubbing. Auscultation reveals clear lung fields, and the cardiac examination shows a right ventricular lift, a normal 1st heart sound, and a single 2nd sound. A grade II/VI systolic ejection murmur is heard at the left sternal border in the 3rd intercostal space. There is no edema or hepatomegaly, and the peripheral pulses are normal.

ADDITIONAL DATA

The chest x-ray shows the heart size is normal, although right heart enlargement is noted on the lateral view (loss of retrosternal clear space). The ECG shows right axis deviation, right ventricular hypertrophy and an intraventricular conduction delay to the right. A complete blood count shows a hemoglobin of 22.3 g/dl and hemotocrit of 66%.

QUESTIONS

1. What is the diagnosis?
2. What pathophysiologic mechanisms explain these symptoms?
3. What would you expect to see on an echocardiogram?
4. What is the significance of the elevated hemoglobin and hematocrit?
5. Is cardiac catheterization indicated?
6. Is surgery indicated?

ANSWERS

1. Tetralogy of Fallot. The characteristic features are progressive cyanosis, spells which improve with squatting, a single S2, right ventricular hypertrophy and a boot-shaped heart on chest x-ray (small pulmonary artery and apex tipped up). The most common cardiac lesion producing cyanosis in an infant is transposition of the great arteries, whereas over the age of 5 tetralogy is the most common etiology. Other causes of cyanotic congenital heart disease in the adult include pulmonic atresia with VSD, pulmonic stenosis with ASD, and VSD, PDA or ASD with Eisenmenger's reaction. Less commonly encountered is Ebstein's anomaly with ASD.

2. The 4 features of tetralogy of Fallot include: (1) nonrestrictive ventricular septal defect, (2) obstruction to right ventricular (RV) outflow (infundibular stenosis), (3) RV hypertrophy, and (4) "overriding aorta." Progressive cyanosis is explained by worsening of the infundibular stenosis, resulting in an increased right-to-left shunt. Exercise lowers peripheral vascular resistance and increases right-to-left shunting. This decreases the pulmonary flow at a time when oxygen demands are actually increased. Posturing such as squatting, leg-crossing and lying down help alleviate these symptoms.

3. The echocardiogram shows aortic enlargement, aortic-septal discontinuity, and aortic overriding of the ventricular septum. Saline contrast injection in a peripheral vein shows a cloud of echos in the left ventricle, confirming the right-to-left shunt.

4. The chronic hypoxemia from right-to-left shunting is a stimulus to increased erythropoietin production resulting in polycythemia. Frequently, the hematocrit can exceed 60-65% with a result of increased blood viscosity. This is often associated with headaches and, in unfortunate cases, bleeding, intravascular thromboses and thrombotic strokes. Phlebotomy is indicated in this patient with symptoms of hyperviscosity.

5. Cardiac catheterization is indicated to confirm the diagnosis, assess the magnitude of the shunt, and evaluate the anatomic features of the RV outflow, pulmonic valve, pulmonary arteries and coronary arteries.

6. If anatomically feasible, repair should be undertaken. This involves right infundibulectomy, pulmonary valvulotomy, patch closure of the ventricular septal defect, and a right ventricular outflow patch.

PEARLS

1.  Tetralogy of Fallot is the most common cause of cyanotic congenital heart disease in the adult.
2.  The majority of patients with tetralogy of Fallot are of slight stature.
3.  Several central nervous system complications can be associated with this syndrome, including brain damage and mental retardation secondary to severe hypoxic spells, brain abscess, cerebral embolism and sinus venous thrombosis.
4.  Patients with tetralogy of Fallot rarely live into late adulthood without surgical repair.

PITFALLS

1.  Pregnancy is not well tolerated and must be discouraged in women with unrepaired tetralogy.
2.  Ventricular ectopy in postoperative patients with tetralogy of Fallot is a common finding.  When the ectopy is associated with residual hemodynamic abnormalities, there is an increased risk of sudden death.
3.  Complete heart block may occur in the early and late postoperative periods following surgical repair of tetralogy of Fallot.

REFERENCES

Abraham KA, Cherian G, Rao VD, et al:  Tetralogy of Fallot in adults:  A report of 147 patients.  Am J Med 66:811, 1979.
Bertranoc EG, Blackstone EH, Hazelrig JB, et al:  Life expectancy without surgery in tetralogy of Fallot.  Am J Cardiol 43:458, 1978.
Borow KM, Green LH, Castaneda AR, Kean JF:  Left ventricular function after repair of tetralogy of Fallot and its relationship to age at surgery.  Circulation 61:1150, 1980.
Higgins CB, Mulden DG:  Tetralogy of Fallot in the adult.  Am J Med 29:837, 1972.
Klotz NM, Blackstone EH, Kirklin JW, et al:  Late survival and symptoms after repair of tetralogy of Fallot.  Circulation 65:403, 1982.
Perloff JK:  The Clinical Recognition of Congenital Heart Disease. Philadelphia, WB Saunders, 1987.
Wessel KU, Bostanier CK, Pearl MK, et al:  Prognostic significance of

arrhythmia in tetralogy of Fallot after intracardiac repair.   Am J
Cardiol 46:843, 1980.

## CASE 23: CHEST PAIN IN A YOUNG MAN

HISTORY

A 24-year-old male graduate student presents with 2 days of moderately severe chest pain--a sharp sensation which is exacerbated by a deep breath or coughing. He is more comfortable sitting up than lying supine. He has been healthy previously and denies any systemic illnesses. He takes no medication and has never had any cardiovascular symptoms in the past. There is no history of trauma to the chest. There is no family history of heart disease, and the patient has no risk factors for coronary artery disease.

EXAMINATION

Physical examination reveals a well-developed young male with a blood pressure of 110/60, respirations of 14 and a pulse rate of 85. There is no jugular venous distension. He has a regular rate and rhythm. There is a 2-component friction rub, but no murmur is heard. The rest of the examination is normal.

The ECG is shown below:

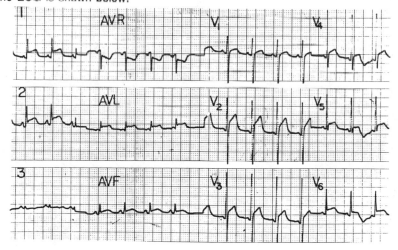

INTERPRETATION OF ECG: Diffuse ST segment elevation; the PR segments are depressed in several leads.

QUESTIONS

1. What is the diagnosis?
2. What is the most likely etiology of this problem?
3. What laboratory tests might be of value in assessing this problem?
4. What therapy would you recommend?

ANSWERS

1. Acute pericarditis.
2. In most cases of pericarditis the etiology is not established. Many cases are preceded by a viral syndrome, and infectious viral pericarditis is then diagnosed. The most likely viruses include coxsackie, echo, influenza and herpes.
3. A complete blood count may suggest an infection. An erythrocyte sedimentation rate (ESR) will usually be elevated and can help in following the course and assessing the response to therapy. Other serologic tests, such as acute and chronic viral titers, antinuclear antibody, rheumatoid factor and hepatitis antigen, may be helpful in establishing a diagnosis when suggested clinically. A blood urea nitrogen and creatinine may be obtained to exclude uremic pericarditis.
4. Therapy should be directed at the underlying etiology if a treatable cause can be found. The chest pain may be relieved by salicylates or nonsteroidal anti-inflammatory drugs. If the pain is severe, a short course of corticosteroid therapy may be necessary for symptomatic relief.

PEARLS

1. Since the pain of pericarditis may be aggravated by inspiration, many patients will complain of shortness of breath.
2. The friction rub is the most common physical finding in pericarditis and is usually triphasic in character: a systolic component during ventricular systole, an early diastolic component occurring during the early phase of ventricular filling, and a presystolic component synchronous with atrial systole.
3. Malignant tumors may cause pericarditis; the most common tumors metastatic to the pericardium are from the breast or lung. Other tumors with a significant incidence of metastasis to the pericardium include lymphoma, leukemia and melanoma.
4. Rheumatoid arthritis, systemic lupus, scleroderma, polyarteritis and other connective tissue disorders can cause pericarditis. Drug-induced lupus syndrome due to procainamide, hydralazine, isoniazid or diphenylhydantoin should also be considered.
5. Pericarditis may occur within the 1st week after a transmural myocardial infarction. This is distinct from Dressler's syndrome of

fever, pericarditis and pleuritis, which occurs weeks to months after an infarction and may have an immunologic basis.

## PITFALLS

1. An echocardiogram is often ordered in this setting to look for a pericardial effusion. Many patients with pericarditis have normal echocardiograms without a pericardial effusion.
2. Pericardiocentesis is rarely indicated as a diagnostic procedure and is generally only indicated when cardiac tamponade is present.
3. The ECG in pericarditis is variable and may be seen in any of its 4 phases: (1) ST segment elevation, (2) return of ST segments to baseline, (3) T wave inversions, and (4) return to normal.
4. Acute ECG changes are often difficult to differentiate from the early repolarization syndrome (a normal variant).

## REFERENCES

Baltwood CM, Shah PM: The pericardium in health and disease. Curr Probl Cardiol 9:9, 1984.

Shabetai R: The pericardium: An essay on some recent developments. Am J Cardiol 42:1036, 1978.

Surawicz B, Lasseter KC: Electrocardiogram in pericarditis. Am J Cardiol 26:471, 1970.

## CASE 24: LUNG CANCER AND CARDIOMEGALY

HISTORY

A 50-year-old school administrator is admitted for progressive shortness of breath and orthopnea of 2 weeks duration. One year ago she was found to have adenocarcinoma of the right lung with extensive involvement of mediastinal lymph nodes and has undergone 2 chemotherapeutic trials without apparent benefit. She denies chest pain, fever, chills or hemoptysis. There is no history of heart disease. She has been given diuretics for the past 2 days by her family doctor without improvement in her breathing.

EXAMINATION

The patient is a thin, chronically ill woman in moderate respiratory distress, sitting upright. Heart rate is 110; blood pressure is 98/68 (with 20 mm of paradox); temperature is 37oC; respirations are 28. The neck veins are elevated to the angle of the jaw; the peripheral pulse is regular but nearly disappears with inspiration. There is dullness to percussion at both lung bases, but there are no rales or wheezes. The heart tones are distant; no gallop, murmur or rub is heard. The liver edge is 8 cm below the right costal margin. There is prominent clubbing of the fingers and toes but no peripheral edema.

ADDITIONAL DATA

The chest radiograph shows cardiomegaly, which is new since 1 month ago, bilateral pleural effusions and a right hilar mass. The hemoglobin is 9.5 mg/dl; the white cell count is 9,400 with normal differential. Arterial blood gases on room air show: $pO_2$ = 69; $pCO_2$ = 21; and pH = 7.50.

CLUES FROM THE ECHOCARDIOGRAM AND RHYTHM STRIP:

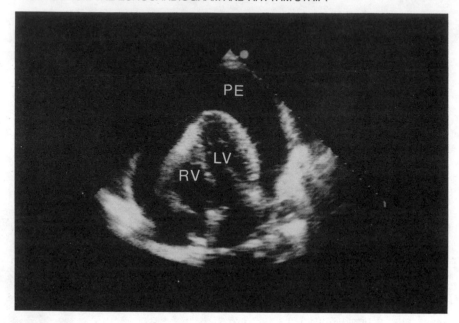

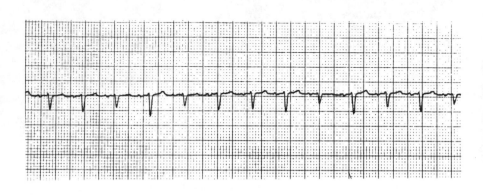

INTERPRETATION OF ECHOCARDIOGRAM: This is an apical 4-chamber view which shows a large pericardial effusion (PE). LV = left ventricle; RV = right ventricle.

INTERPRETATION OF RHYTHM STRIP: Sinus rhythm with electrical alternans.

QUESTIONS

1. What is the cause of this woman's dyspnea, hypotension and tachycardia?
2. What are common etiologies of this clinical problem?
3. What are the malignancies that most often result in this problem?
4. What would you expect to be the effect of diuretics in this patient?
5. What treatment would you institute?
6. What is her prognosis?

ANSWERS

1. Pericardial tamponade. Characteristic features are the combination of pulsus paradoxus and the echocardiographic findings of a large pericardial effusion with early diastolic collapse of the right ventricle.
2. In most large series, malignancies account for the greatest number of cases. Other etiologies include radiation-induced, viral, renal failure, congestive heart failure, collagen vascular diseases, and bacterial infections.
3. Carcinoma of the lung and breast are the most common. Other malignancies that affect the pericardium include melanoma, leukemia and lymphoma.
4. Tamponade results from the limitations to cardiac filling from increased intrapericardial pressure within the closed pericardial space. Diuresis and reduction in venous return may aggravate the condition and cause severe hypotension and collapse.
5. Initial treatment includes intravenous fluid challenge and prompt removal of fluid from the pericardial space (pericardiocentesis). Reaccumulation of fluid may be prevented by the installation of a sclerosing substance (e.g., tetracycline, bleomycin), by radiation therapy, or by a surgical procedure such as a pericardial window or pericardiectomy.
6. The prognosis for patients with malignant pericardial effusion and tamponade is guarded, and average survival is approximately 3-6 months.

PEARLS

1. The rate of accumulation, not necessarily the size of the effusion, is the most important factor in determining the occurrence of tamponade; the sudden accumulation of as little as 100 cc of fluid may cause cardiac compression, whereas the gradual buildup of as much as 2 liters may have no hemodynamic consequences.
2. In most cases of clinically significant tamponade, pulsus paradoxus can be appreciated by palpation.
3. Early diastolic collapse of the right atrium and ventricle are relatively sensitive and specific echocardiographic signs of tamponade which generally precede low cardiac output and pulsus

paradoxus.

4. Electrical alternans, i.e., alternating QRS axis due to swinging of the heart in the pericardial fluid, is strongly suggestive of pericardial effusion and often accompanies cardiac tamponade.

5. The short-term survival in cardiac tamponade depends on prompt diagnosis and therapy of cardiac compression; the long-term survival is determined by the underlying condition resulting in the pericardial effusion.

## PITFALLS

1. The presence of pulsus paradoxus may be masked when the cardiac rhythm is irregular, such as with atrial fibrillation.

2. Kussmaul's sign, i.e., the increase in neck vein pressure with inspiration, is a feature of cardiac constriction due to a rigid pericardium and is not generally seen in the elastic cardiac compression with effusion and tamponade.

3. Patients with uremic pericarditis and impending tamponade tolerate hemodialysis poorly, because of the rapid fluid changes that may result in inadequate filling volumes.

4. Pulsus paradoxus may disappear in severe cardiac tamponade.

## REFERENCES

Boltwood CM Jr, Shah PM: The pericardium in health and disease. Curr Probl Cardiol 9:1, 1984.

Hancock EW: Cardiac tamponade. Med Clin North Am 63:223, 1979.

Kralstein J, Frishman W: Malignant pericardial disease: Diagnosis and treatment. Am Heart J 113:785, 1987.

Markiewicz W, Borovik R, Ecker S: Cardiac tamponade in medical patients: Treatment and prognosis in the echocardiographic era. Am Heart J 111:1138, 1986.

McGregor M: Pulsus paradoxus. N Engl J Med 301:480, 1979.

## CASE 25: CHRONIC ARTHRITIS AND RIGHT-SIDED HEART FAILURE

HISTORY

A 46-year-old teacher presents with a 1-year history of chronic fatigue, intermittent atypical chest pain, a nonproductive cough and a 15-pound weight loss. He has chronic rheumatoid arthritis with olecranon nodules, moderate synovitis and a rheumatoid factor of 1:512. Recently he has noted dyspnea, moderate ankle edema, occasional paroxysmal nocturnal dyspnea, and increasing abdominal girth. There is no prior history of organic heart disease. He is a nonsmoker.

EXAMINATION

The physical examination reveals an asthenic male without clubbing or cyanosis. Blood pressure is 100/75; heart rate is 110. The lung fields are clear to auscultation and percussion. There is jugular venous distension to 10 cm of $H_2O$ with an inspiratory increase in pressure and rapid descent during diastole. The heart sounds are decreased, and a diastolic sound is heard at the lower left sternal border, just after S2. The abdomen is mildly distended, with moderate hepatomegaly and a fluid wave, and mild ankle edema is also present.

ADDITIONAL DATA

The chest x-ray shows mild cardiomegaly with pulmonary vascular redistribution and small bilateral pleural effusions. The ECG shows a low-voltage QRS with nonspecific ST and T wave abnormalities. The echocardiogram shows a small pericardial effusion with an atrial systolic notch and abnormal diastolic flattening of the left ventricular posterior wall.

## QUESTIONS

1. What is the diagnosis? What are the most common etiologies of this problem?
2. What drugs have been implicated in this problem?
3. What aspects of the physical examination are characteristic of cardiac constriction and help to differentiate it from cardiac tamponade?
4. How is the echocardiogram helpful in this diagnosis?
5. What confirmatory studies are performed before therapy can be completed?
6. What therapy is recommended for this entity?

ANSWERS

1.  Constrictive pericarditis.  Prior to the age of antimicrobial therapy, tuberculosis was the most common cause of constrictive pericarditis. Recent studies show that an increasing number of patients present without an apparent cause; some of these may have suffered previous episodes of "viral" or idiopathic pericarditis.  Prior heart surgery, uremia, neoplasms and connective tissue disease (especially rheumatoid arthritis) represent other causes of this rare disease.

2.  Drugs implicated in causing constrictive pericarditis include hydralazine, procainamide and methysergide.

3.  The clinical features of "compressive" pericardial disease may overlap; however, characteristic of constrictive pericarditis is the presence of Kussmaul's sign (inspiratory increase in jugular venous pressure), a prominent Y descent and a pericardial knock (following S2).  Although pulsus paradoxus is characteristic of cardiac tamponade, it may be present with constriction (30% of cases) but usually will not exceed 15 mm.

4.  Although the echocardiogram is a critical element in the work-up, the findings may be subtle and overlap with other pathologic conditions. A thickened pericardium may be detected, usually noted as dense parallel echos from the visceral and parietal pericardium separated by a small effusion. (Fast contrast tomography and magnetic resonance imaging may be preferred modalities to detect thickening.)

5.  Cardiac catheterization is useful to clarify the hemodynamic profile and the severity of the lesion.  The typical findings include equalization of the right atrial, right ventricular end-diastolic, pulmonary artery diastolic, pulmonary capillary wedge, and left ventricular end-diastolic pressures.  The ventricular pressure tracings show a "dip and plateau" pattern, and the atrial tracings, an "M" or "W" pattern with a prominent Y descent.

6.  Pericardiectomy is the treatment of choice for constrictive pericarditis.  Antituberculous therapy must be instituted prior to surgery if tuberculosis is the cause of the constrictive pericarditis.

PEARLS

1.  Pericardial constriction may develop as early as 3 months or as late as several years following mediastinal radiation.

2.  Episodic, recurrent "idiopathic" pericarditis may be the cause of

constrictive pericarditis in up to 20% of patients.

3. The chest x-ray may show pericardial calcification, which is best detected on the lateral view and may be seen in the atrioventricular groove or along the anterior or inferior surfaces of the right ventricle.

## PITFALLS

1. Restrictive cardiomyopathies due to amyloidosis, hemochromatosis or eosinophilic endomyocardial fibrosis may present in a similar fashion and may have the same hemodynamic characteristics as constrictive disease. Endomyocardial biopsy may be helpful in distinguishing between restrictive and constrictive disease. Rarely, thoracotomy is performed as a final effort to clarify the etiology and provide therapy in constrictive pericarditis.

2. Cardiac catheterization may not show the characteristic hemodynamic abnormalities if volume depletion is present. Administration of a saline challenge (i.e., 1 liter of normal saline solution) may bring out the expected findings.

3. Surgical mortality for pericardiectomy may be as high as 4-6% and cannot be recommended without conclusive noninvasive and invasive data.

4. Symptoms may be subacute, vague, slowly progressive with subtle abnormalities, and mistaken for a psychosomatic illness.

## REFERENCES

Applefeld MM, Cold JF, Pollock SH, et al: The late appearance of chronic pericardial disease in patients treated by radiotherapy for Hodgkin's disease. Ann Intern Med 94:338, 1981.

Candell-Riera J, Garcia del Castillo H, Permanyer-Miralda G, et al: Echo features of the interventricular septum in chronic constrictive pericarditis. Circulation 57:1154, 1978.

Cohen MV, Greenberg MA: Constrictive pericarditis: Early and late complications of cardiac surgery. Am J Cardiol 43:657, 1979.

Hirschmann JV: Pericardial constriction. Am Heart J 96:110, 1978.

Howard EJ, Maier H: Constrictive pericarditis following acute coxsackie viral pericarditis. Am Heart J 75:247, 1968.

Ikram H, Banin SO, Makey AR: Clinical features of nontuberculous constricted pericarditis.   Thorax 29:204, 1974.

Nicholson WJ, Cobbs BW, Franch RH, et al:   Early diastolic sound of constrictive pericarditis.   Am J Cardiol 45:378, 1980.

Schnittger I, Bowden RE, Abrams J, et al:   Echocardiography:   Pericardial thickening and constrictive pericarditis.   Am J Cardiol 42:388, 1978.

## CASE 26: SUDDEN COLLAPSE WITH CARDIAC ARREST

CLINICAL PRESENTATION

A 59-year-old retired railroad worker collapses in his front yard during a casual talk with his neighbor. Cardiopulmonary resuscitation is instituted immediately, and the paramedics are called. Upon arrival, the paramedics find the patient to be unresponsive, with no pulse and no spontaneous respirations.

The patient has no previous known cardiac disease. He is a nonsmoker, and there is no history of diabetes or hypertension. A routine company physical 3 years ago revealed a cholesterol level of 272 mg/dl. An ECG at that time showed some notching of the QRS in the inferior leads and 2 premature ventricular contractions.

The patient's rhythm at the time of the paramedics' arrival is shown below:

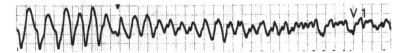

QUESTIONS

1. What is the rhythm on the above strip?
2. What definitive therapy should be administered by the paramedics?
3. What is the most likely etiology of this sudden death episode? Is it likely that the patient is having a myocardial infarction?
4. Assuming successful resuscitation from this event, what is the likelihood of a recurrence in the next year?
5. What management program for this sudden cardiac death survivor should be considered?

ANSWERS

1. Ventricular fibrillation.
2. Electrical defibrillation with 200-300 watt-seconds.
3. Coronary artery disease is by far the most common cause of sudden death. Sudden death should not be equated with "a massive heart attack," since most victims have not suffered a myocardial infarction.
4. Patients who develop ventricular fibrillation which is not the direct result of an acute myocardial infarction have a 30-35% recurrence rate within 12 months if untreated.
5. An aggressive management program is warranted. Electrophysiologic testing with programmed electrical stimulation should be considered. Drug therapy is then judged by its ability to suppress ventricular tachycardia or fibrillation on repeat testing. An alternative, noninvasive approach using exercise testing and ambulatory monitoring involves empiric drug therapy with the goal of near-complete (>85%) suppression of the ventricular ectopy. Certain patients who fail drug therapy may respond to coronary bypass surgery or coronary angioplasty, presumably because their ectopy is ischemic in origin. Other therapeutic modalities include the placement of an automatic implantable defibrillator or ablative techniques.

PEARLS

1. Sudden cardiac death is the leading cause of death in the United States, claiming approximately 400,000 victims annually.
2. Sudden death may be the first indication of clinical heart disease; approximately 25% of victims have had no prior symptoms of heart disease.
3. The majority of sudden cardiac death victims do not collapse during vigorous activity.

PITFALLS

1. There is no universally accepted definition of sudden cardiac death. When defined as death within 24 hours of the onset of acute symptoms, approximately 60% of cases can be ascribed to coronary artery disease (CAD). When defined as death within an hour of the

onset of symptoms, 91% of cases can be attributed to CAD.

2. It is unproven that in the general population suppression of premature ventricular complexes protects against sudden cardiac death.
3. Routine risk factors for coronary artery disease do not define a special subset of patients prone to sudden cardiac death.
4. Antiarrhythmic drugs may aggravate an individual patient's arrhythmia ("proarrhythmic effect").
5. Certain iatrogenic misadventures may precipitate sudden cardiac death. Some of these include: digitalis toxicity, kaliuretic diuretics, liquid protein diets, tricyclic antidepressant and phenothiazine overdose and rarely, inappropriate pacemaker implants.
6. Sometimes it is difficult to determine whether ventricular fibrillation resulted from a myocardial infarction or whether myocardial necrosis occurred as a result of the cardiac arrest.

REFERENCES

Bigger JT, Roiffol JA, Levelli FD, et al: Sensitivity, specificity, and reproducibility of programmed ventricular stimulation. Circulation 73:l1, 1986.

Cobb LA, Werner JA, Trobough GB: Sudden cardiac death: I. A decade's experience with out-of-hospital resuscitation. Mod Concepts Cardiovasc Dis 49:31, 1980.

Lown B: Sudden cardiac death: The major challenge confronting contemporary cardiology. Am J Cardiol 43:313, 1979.

Mirowski M, Reid PR, Mower MM, et al: Termination of malignant ventricular arrhythmias with an implanted automatic defibrillator in human beings. N Engl J Med 303:322, 1980.

## CASE 27: LIGHTHEADEDNESS AND A WIDE QRS TACHYCARDIA

HISTORY

A 68-year-old retired insurance executive comes to the emergency room complaining of lightheadedness of 2 hours duration. He has a known history of anterior wall myocardial infarction which occurred 4 years ago, occasional premature ventricular contractions (PVC's), and a left ventricular ejection fraction of 36% as determined by nuclear ventriculography. He denies recent angina pectoris, and there is no history of previous palpitations or syncope. He is taking no medications.

EXAMINATION

This is a mildly obese male who is anxious and in no respiratory distress. Heart rate is 150 and regular; blood pressure is 100/60 (his usual BP is 130/80). The jugular pulsation shows Intermittent and prominent A waves; the lungs reveal bibasilar crackles. The left ventricular (LV) impulse is in the 6th intercostal space in the anterior axillary line; the 1st heart sound is variable. No murmurs or gallops are appreciated.

CLUE FROM THE ECG

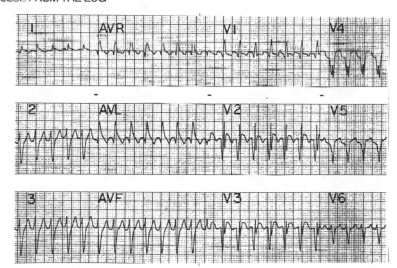

QUESTIONS

1. What is the differential diagnosis of "wide QRS complex" tachycardia?
2. What diagnosis is most likely in this case, as suggested by the ECG?
3. How might this be confirmed?
4. What treatment would you initiate?
5. What is the prognostic significance of the dysrhythmia in this patient with known coronary artery disease?
6. What further evaluation should be considered to assess the response to therapy?

ANSWERS

1. Wide QRS tachycardia may be supraventricular tachycardia (SVT) with aberrant conduction due to bundle branch block or to conduction via an accessory pathway. However, wide QRS tachycardia is most commonly ventricular tachycardia (VT).
2. The width of the QRS complex (greater than 0.14 second), the biphasic presence of atrioventricular (AV) dissociation, left axis, and the complex in lead V1 strongly suggest that this is VT.
3. Slowing the rhythm with medication such as lidocaine or procainamide might help to confirm the presence of AV dissociation, which essentially only occurs with VT. Esophageal or atrial recordings are occasionally helpful to show atrial activity that may not otherwise be seen during the tachycardia. The definitive test in the diagnosis of VT is electrophysiologic study.
4. Prompt electrical cardioversion should be considered if the rhythm does not respond within a few minutes to intravenous loading with either lidocaine or procainamide. Overdrive pacing with a temporary ventricular electrode is another method of cardioversion; however, there is a possibility that overdrive pacing may accelerate the tachycardia.
5. Patients with VT and underlying ischemic heart disease have a high mortality, and aggressive therapy with antiarrhythmic medication is warranted.
6. Ventricular tachycardia in this patient is a life-threatening arrhythmia; many authors would recommend electrophysiologic testing in an attempt to induce the rhythm under controlled conditions in order to find a medical regimen that would then prevent induction. Survival is improved in patients who are no longer inducible on medication.

PEARLS

1. The vast majority of tachyarrhythmias with a QRS complex width greater than 0.14 second (140 msec) are ventricular in origin.
2. Monophasic or biphasic QRS complexes in lead V1 are suggestive of VT, whereas triphasic complexes (rSr′) are more commonly seen with supraventricular tachycardia with aberrant conduction.
3. Intracardiac electrograms, which can be obtained by using a temporary pacing electrode, may be helpful in demonstrating

atrioventricular dissociation and thus the presence of VT.

4.   An irregular, wide QRS tachycardia with a rate greater than 220 beats/minute should suggest the possibility of atrial fibrillation with conduction over an accessory (bypass) pathway, such as in the Wolff-Parkinson-White (WPW) syndrome.

PITFALLS

1.   Some patients may tolerate VT without syncope or hypotension; the presence of only mild symptoms does not exclude the diagnosis of VT.
2.   It may be impossible to reliably distinguish VT from SVT with aberrancy by physical examination and the 12-lead ECG; invasive testing using electrophysiologic techniques may be required.
3.   Ventriculoatrial conduction (without AV dissociation) occurs in up to 1/3 of cases of VT, and thus the absence of AV dissociation may not be helpful in the diagnosis of wide QRS tachycardia.
4.   Although the morphology of the QRS complex in wide QRS tachycardia may be helpful in distinguishing SVT with aberrancy from VT, these criteria are unreliable in the presence of accessory pathways, such as in WPW syndrome.

REFERENCES

Horowitz LN, Spielman SR, Greenspan AM, Josephson ME:   Role of programmed stimulation in assessing vulnerability to ventricular arrhythmias.   Am Heart J 103:604, 1982.

Kienzle MG, Doherty JU, Marcus NH, et al:   When do electrophysiologic studies benefit arrhythmia patients?   J Cardiovasc Med 1:41, 1984.

Swerdlow CD, Winkle RA, Mason JW:   Determinants of survival in patients with ventricular tachyarrhythmias.   N Engl J Med 308:1436, 1983.

Wellens HJJ, Bar FWHM, Tie KI:   The value of the electrocardiogram in the differential diagnosis of a tachycardia with a widened QRS complex.   Am J Med 64:27, 1978.

Wellens HJJ, Brugada P, Stevenson WG:   Programmed electrical stimulation of the heart in patients with life-threatening ventricular arrhythmias:   What is the significance of induced arrhythmias and what is the correct stimulation protocol?   Circulation 72:1, 1985

## CASE 28: IRREGULAR HEART POUNDING IN A HEALTHY MAN

HISTORY

A 65-year-old electrician presents to the emergency room with a 1-day history of rapid heart pounding and fatigue. He has had no complaints of chest pain, dyspnea or syncope. He had an uncomplicated myocardial infarction 8 years ago and has had no angina since that time. He has a history of borderline high blood pressure and elevated cholesterol; he had smoked 1 pack of cigarettes per day but stopped smoking after his heart attack.

EXAMINATION

Physical examination reveals a well-developed, well-nourished male in no acute distress, with a blood pressure of 140/90, a rapid irregular pulse of 160, and respirations of 12/minute. His cardiac examination reveals an irregular rhythm. There is no evidence of cardiac enlargement. The heart sounds are normal, and there are no systolic or diastolic murmurs. The remainder of his examination is unremarkable.

This patient's ECG is shown below:

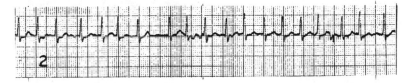

QUESTIONS

1. What is the rhythm?
2. What is the most likely etiology of this problem?
3. Several clinical questions should be answered before approaching the therapy for this problem:
   a. How is the patient tolerating the rhythm?
   b. Is this an acute or chronic problem?
   c. What is the size of the left atrium?
   d. What is the likelihood that the patient will revert to sinus rhythm?
4. What therapy should be instituted?
5. When should electrical cardioversion be considered?

ANSWERS

1. Atrial fibrillation.
2. The most likely cause of atrial fibrillation in this case (and the most common cause in general) is coronary artery disease. Other etiologies include valvular heart disease (especially mitral valve disease), cardiomyopathy, hypertension, pericarditis, chronic obstructive pulmonary disease and hyperthyroidism.
3. In this case, the patient is tolerating the rhythm. well, and this appears to be a recent problem. The echocardiogram reveals a normal-sized left atrium. These facts suggest that the patient will likely revert to sinus rhythm with therapy.
4. Initial therapy would include digoxin to slow the ventricular rate response to less than 100 beats/minute. Since the goal in this patient is to attempt medical cardioversion, an atrial antiarrhythmic such as quinidine should be added after the rate is slowed with digoxin.
5. If the patient's rhythm does not revert to sinus rhythm within a short period, anticoagulation (coumadin) should be started and continued for 3 weeks, and then electrical cardioversion attempted. Digoxin is usually stopped for 1-2 days prior to the procedure. Most patients can be sedated with diazepam or given a very short-acting barbiturate for anesthesia, and the electrical cardioversion done with 200-300 watt-seconds. In most cases, cardioversion is achieved after 1 or 2 electrical shocks. If 3 shocks are given and the patient remains in atrial fibrillation, further attempts are generally not warranted.

PEARLS

1. Atrial fibrillation does occur in the absence of overt cardiovascular disease or precipitating illness. This is known as lone atrial fibrillation and occurs in approximately 3% of all patients with atrial fibrillation.
2. Atrial fibrillation is a common arrhythmia after open heart surgery, especially with bypass surgery patients. Generally, this is well tolerated, is short lived, and can be treated with digitalis to slow the ventricular response rate. Electrical cardioversion is usually not necessary, as most patients will revert back to sinus rhythm within 24-48 hours. The mechanism of atrial fibrillation in

this setting is thought to be due to pericardial irritation or to mechanical atrial manipulation at the time of surgery.

3. Patients with chronic atrial fibrillation are at increased risk of embolic stroke, and this risk increases directly with the duration of atrial fibrillation. This risk is highest in rheumatic mitral valve disease patients and in those with ischemic heart disease.

## PITFALLS

1. Patients with hypertrophic cardiomyopathy do not tolerate atrial fibrillation well; therefore, vigorous efforts should be made to maintain sinus rhythm in this subgroup.
2. Patients who present with atrial fibrillation and ventricular rates of less than 100 beats/minute on no drug therapy should be suspected of having conduction tissue disease involving the AV node. Caution should be taken in this subset when considering digitalis, beta blockers, calcium blockers or electrical cardioversion. Some will require pacemakers if symptomatic slow rates are part of the "tachy-brady" syndrome.
3. The role of anticoagulation prior to cardioversion is somewhat controversial. Most authorities agree that anticoagulation is indicated in patients with high risk of emboli, such as those with mitral stenosis, prosthetic mitral valve, recurrent emboli or cardiomegaly.

## REFERENCES

Hinton RC, Kistler JP, Fallon JT, et al: Influence of etiology of atrial fibrillation on incidence of systemic embolization. Am J Cardiol 40:509, 1977.

Kopecky SL, Gersh BJ, Phil D, et al: The natural history of lone atrial fibrillation: A population-based study over 3 decades. N Engl J Med 317:669, 1987.

Mancini GBJ, Goldberger AL: Cardioversion of atrial fibrillation: Consideration of embolization, anticoagulation, prophylactic pacemaker and long-term success. Am Heart J 104:617, 1982.

## CASE 29: VENTRICULAR FIBRILLATION IN THE CORONARY CARE UNIT

HISTORY

A 62-year-old construction worker has the onset of ventricular fibrillation 2 days following admission to the coronary care unit (CCU). He is promptly defibrillated by the nursing staff, and within a short time he is awake and alert. He denies chest pain, lightheadedness or shortness of breath and does not remember any premonitory symptoms. The patient had been admitted to the CCU when frequent and complex premature ventricular beats were noted by his physician on a routine office visit. Quinidine sulfate 300 mg every 6 hours was begun the day of admission. He has known coronary artery disease with stable angina pectoris occurring with moderate exertion, for which he takes propranolol and occasional sublingual nitroglycerin.

EXAMINATION

Physical examination reveals an alert middle-aged man in no acute distress. His pulse is 84 with frequent premature beats and couplets; blood pressure is 138/76. There is no jugular venous distension, and the carotid upstroke is normal. Auscultation of the heart and lungs reveals no abnormalities.

The rhythm strip just prior to the time of his cardiac arrest is shown below:

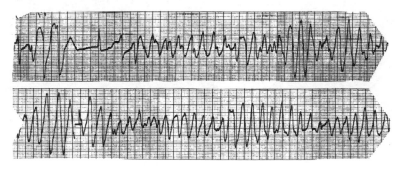

QUESTIONS

1.   What does the rhythm strip show?
2.   What is the most likely precipitating factor?
3.   In what other settings is this dysrhythmia seen?
4.   How would you treat this patient?

ANSWERS

1. Torsades de pointes ("twisting of the points") is a polymorphous ventricular tachycardia in which the peaks of the QRS appear to twist around the isoelectric line. The rhythm is characteristically initiated by a late-cycle premature ventricular contraction (PVC), often exhibits a warm-up phenomenon with frequent couplets and triplets, and may degenerate into ventricular fibrillation.

2. The vast majority of cases of torsades de pointes in adults occurs in the setting of therapy with the type IA antiarrhythmic agents-- quinidine, disopyramide and procainamide. Dramatic and idiosyncratic prolongation of the QT interval (to QTc > 0.50) occurs in 0.5-8% of patients treated with quinidine; a subset of these patients will develop torsades de pointes.

3. Torsades de pointes is seen in other settings, including complete or high-grade AV block, tricyclic antidepressant or phenothiazine overdose, hypokalemia or hypomagnesemia, liquid protein diets, and the congenital long QT syndrome (LQTS). QT prolongation is seen with all of the above and is thought to be a necessary precondition for the development of torsades de pointes.

4. Withdrawal of the offending agent (quinidine, in this case) and avoidance of the other type IA agents associated with QT prolongation are indicated. Bretylium or lidocaine may be tried initially, but the definitive acute treatment is overdrive pacing (preferably atrial), which will generally suppress the arrhythmia. An isoproterenol infusion may be used cautiously to increase the sinus rate if pacing is not immediately available. Magnesium given intravenously has also been used with some success.

PEARLS

1. Torsades de pointes is the culprit rhythm in cases of "quinidine syncope."

2. QT prolongation and abnormal U waves are markers for increased "dispersion of repolarization." This inhomogeneity of refractoriness of the ventricular myocardium is thought by some to be a necessary substrate for torsades.

3. Hypocalcemia causes QT prolongation by lengthening the isoelectric ST segment; this does not increase the dispersion of refractoriness

in the ventricle and is not a cause of torsades.

4. Dramatic QT prolongation occurs commonly following cardiac surgery and in 30% of patients with subarachnoid hemorrhage. However, despite the same degree of QT prolongation as seen in this patient, torsades de pointes is distinctly uncommon in these 2 settings.

5. The congenital long QT syndrome (LQTS) appears to follow an autosomal recessive inheritance pattern when associated with neurogenic deafness (Jervell and Lange-Nielsen syndrome). The Romano-Ward syndrome is the LQTS without deafness. Treatment with beta blockers, left cervicothoracic sympathectomy, and chronic overdrive atrial pacing has decreased the incidence of syncope and sudden death in these young adults.

6. Polymorphous ventricular tachycardia without QT prolongation does occur and is considered by most to be distinct from torsades. Conventional antiarrhythmic drugs, including quinidine, disopyramide and procainamide, may be used for this type of polymorphous tachycardia.

## PITFALLS

1. The degree of QT prolongation does not correlate with the incidence of torsades de pointes, nor does there appear to be a critical degree of QT prolongation that predisposes to the dysrhythmia.

2. Quinidine in therapeutic doses results in a predictable and dose-related increase in the QT interval that is not associated with torsades. Torsades accompanies an idiosyncratic response to the drug, and these patients usually have normal or low therapeutic levels of the antiarrhythmic.

3. Although isoproterenol may help temporarily stabilize patients with acquired torsades, this drug will commonly worsen the dysrhythmia in patients with the congenital syndrome.

4. Electrophysiologic studies in young adults with the congenital LQTS have been unsuccessful in inducing torsades de pointes and are not recommended in patients with this syndrome.

## REFERENCES

Moss AJ, Schwartz PJ, Crampton RS, et al:  The long QT syndrome:  A prospective international study.  Circulation 71:17, 1985.

Sandor R, Morrison D:   Recognizing drug-induced torsades de pointes tachycardia.  Drug Ther 6:134, 1983.

Schweitzer P, Mark H:  Delayed repolarization syndrome.  Am J Med 75:393, 1983.

Smith W, Gallagher J:   Les torsades de pointes:   An unusual ventricular arrhythmia.  Ann Intern Med 93:578, 1980.

Strasberg B, Sclarovsky S, Erdberg AG, et al:   Procainamide-induced polymorphous ventricular tachycardia.  Am J Cardiol 47:1309, 1981.

Surawicz B, Knoebel S:  Long QT:   Good, bad or indifferent?   J Am Coll Cardiol 4:398, 1984.

## CASE 30: PALPITATIONS IN A HEALTHY YOUNG PHYSICIAN

HISTORY

A 29-year-old male physician notes the onset of intermittent palpitations described as a "flip-flop" and pause. As an avid recreational swimmer and basketball player, he has noticed no such symptoms during activity, nor have any symptoms of dizziness, dysequilibrium or syncope occurred. There is no prior history of a murmur, rheumatic fever, chest pain, shortness of breath, orthopnea or edema. He does not smoke, and there are no other risk factors for coronary artery disease.

EXAMINATION

A muscular male with a blood pressure of 105/70, a heart rate of 64, clear lung fields, and normal jugular venous pulsations and carotid upstroke. No murmur or gallop is present; however, frequent premature beats with a pause are noted.

ADDITIONAL DATA

The ECG is normal, except for frequent premature ventricular complexes (PVC's). The Holter shows frequent PVC's (900/hour) with frequent bigeminy and trigeminy and rare couplets. The exercise test, 18 minutes of a Bruce protocol, is completed with normal heart rate and blood pressure response, with frequent PVC's up to 12 minutes, with resolution at peak exercise and with return in the 3rd minute of recovery.

QUESTIONS

1. What other diagnostic studies would you order?
2. What counseling can you provide concerning prognosis?
3. What therapeutic recommendations can be given?
4. If an episode of syncope suggesting a cardiac etiology were to occur, how would you then proceed?
5. What follow-up do you recommend?

ANSWERS

1. An echocardiogram is useful to exclude underlying structural heart disease, such as valvular or myopathic disease. The presence of one of these conditions may impact on therapy or prognosis.
2. This is a complex issue; however, recent data are encouraging and show no change in longevity when patients with frequent PVC's without evidence of "organic heart disease" are compared with a control population.
3. Therapy is not likely to impact on prognosis, and therefore most would not recommend medical treatment. If the awareness of these frequent PVC's becomes bothersome, a trial of therapy may be indicated, such as the use of a beta blocker.
4. If syncope occurs, a vigorous work-up, possibly including an electrophysiologic study, is indicated.
5. Follow-up is particularly important if cardiovascular symptoms occur. Use of follow-up ambulatory monitoring is controversial and must be individualized.

PEARLS

1. Exclusion of "organic heart disease" is important to help determine prognosis and therapy.
2. PVC's in the setting of coronary artery disease imply a worse prognosis; however, there is no proof that therapy improves survival.
3. Stimulants such as caffeine, decongestants and chocolate may aggravate PVC's in some patients.

PITFALLS

1. "Overtreatment" is to be avoided. Antiarrhythmic drugs have been shown to cause serious dysrhythmias and therefore must be used appropriately.
2. Ventricular ectopy may be associated with noncardiac conditions such as hypokalemia, hypomagnesemia and hypoxemia; the ectopy often disappears with treatment of the underlying condition.

REFERENCES

Brodsky M, Wu D, Denes P, et al: Arrhythmias documented by 24-hour continuous electrocardiographic monitoring in 50 male medical students without apparent heart disease. Am J Cardiol 39:390, 1977.

Fley JL, Kennedy HL: Cardiac arrhythmias in a healthy elderly population: Detection by 24-hour ambulatory electrocardiography. Chest 81:302, 1982.

Kennedy HL, Whitlock JA, Sprague MK, et al: Long-term follow-up of asymptomatic healthy subjects with frequent and complex ventricular ectopy. N Engl J Med 312:193, 1985.

Ruskin JN, McGovern G, Garan H, et al: Antiarrhythmic drugs: A possible cause of out-of-hospital cardiac arrest. N Engl J Med 309:1302, 1983.

Sobotha PA, Mayer JU, Bauernfeind RA, et al: Arrhythmias documented by 24-hour continuous ambulatory electrocardiographic monitoring in young women without apparent heart disease. Am Heart J 101:753, 1981.

Velebit V, Podrid PJ, Lown B, et al: Aggravation and provocation of ventricular arrhythmias by antiarrhythmic drugs. Circulation 65:887, 1982.

## CASE 31: SUDDEN HEART POUNDING

HISTORY

A 28-year-old woman comes to the emergency room 2 hours after the abrupt onset of a rapid heart rate and anterior chest discomfort. Although there has been a history of a heart murmur during pregnancy, she has been healthy without previous symptoms and takes no medications.

EXAMINATION

Physical examination reveals a thin, anxious young woman in no acute distress, with a blood pressure of 110/64 and a heart rate that is regular at 210. Prominent, regular jugular venous pulsations are present. The carotid upstroke is normal, and the lungs are clear. The heart reveals a rapid, regular rate, and no murmur is heard.

The patient's ECG is shown below:

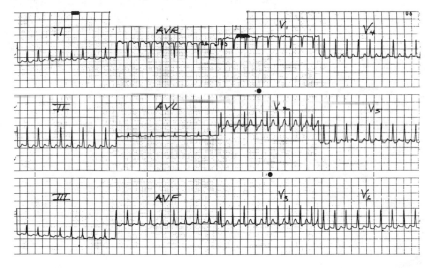

QUESTIONS

1. What is the rhythm disturbance?  What are the most likely underlying heart conditions?
2. What further diagnostic maneuver might help elucidate the nature of the dysrhythmia?
3. What are several possible treatments for this dysrhythmia acutely?
4. What chronic therapy is appropriate?
5. What is this patient's prognosis?

ANSWERS

1.  Paroxysmal supraventricular tachycardia (PSVT).   This general term refers to "narrow QRS" tachycardias that are regular and usually due to a reentry or "circus" mechanism at or above the level of the atrioventricular (AV) node.   Most patients with PSVT have no underlying heart disease.   PSVT is seen with increased frequency in those with mitral valve prolapse, anomalous bypass tracts and various forms of congenital heart disease.
2.  Carotid sinus massage (CSM).   This maneuver causes a reflex stimulation of the vagus nerve that may result in an abrupt termination or slight slowing of PSVT.   By increasing parasympathetic tone to the AV node, CSM may increase AV block and reveal flutter waves when a regular, narrow QRS tachycardia is due to atrial flutter.
3.  Verapamil is now established as the drug of first choice in the acute treatment of PSVT and successfully converts over 90% of patients to sinus rhythm.   Prior to the availability of intravenous verapamil, the short-acting cholinesterase inhibitor edrophonium (Tensilon) and pressor agents were used.
4.  Patients with infrequent episodes of nonsustained PSVT who have no underlying structural heart disease do not require special long-term therapy.   The patient should be taught the Valsalva maneuver to try to break the PSVT at home.   In addition, immersing the face in cold water will elicit the diving reflex and may interrupt the tachycardia.   Chronic therapy to prevent PSVT includes digoxin, beta-blocking agents and oral verapamil.   Medical therapy to prevent PSVT should be reserved for sustained dysrhythmias that necessitate repeated visits to the emergency room or otherwise significantly interfere with the patient's life-style.
5.  Subsequent examination when this patient was in sinus rhythm was entirely within normal limits, as was her chest x-ray and electrocardiogram.   Although she may experience further episodes of PSVT and may possibly require preventive therapy, her prognosis is excellent, and she should be reassured accordingly.

PEARLS

1.  The most common mechanism for PSVT is AV nodal reentry, which is responsible for approximately 60% of cases.

2. P waves are characteristically buried in the QRS complex in PSVT when the mechanism is AV nodal reentry. When P waves are seen following the QRS, in the ST segment, or early in the T wave, one a bypass tract should be suspected as the retrograde limb of the reentrant circuit.

3. The atrial rate in atrial flutter is characteristically 300, and patients usually present with 1:2 conduction and a regular tachycardia at 150 beats/minute.

4. Reentry within the sinus node is an infrequent cause of PSVT and accounts for only 5-10% of "narrow QRS tachycardias." When sinus node reentry is the cause of PSVT, the rate is relatively slow (130-140/minute).

5. Paroxysmal atrial tachycardia (PAT), associated with AV block, is often due to digitalis toxicity and results from abnormally increased automaticity.

6. Anomalous or "bypass" connections between the atrium and ventricle are involved in the reentrant circuits in approximately 20% of cases of PSVT.

PITFALLS

1. Patients with PSVT may have chest pain that is typical of myocardial infarction or ischemia. However, many--if not most--do not have associated coronary artery disease.

2. Commonly, the ECG immediately following conversion to sinus rhythm shows transient ST or T wave changes that are abnormal and suggest ischemia. These abnormalities may be the result of the dysrhythmia or may be secondary to the drug therapy used to convert the rhythm. The ECG usually returns to normal in minutes to hours.

3. Patients with PSVT may present with a rate-related bundle branch block; differentiation of this "wide QRS tachycardia" from ventricular tachycardia may be impossible. In such cases, it is often safer to assume that the rhythm is ventricular and life-threatening. Treatment with lidocaine or procainamide intravenously may be necessary, or direct current cardioversion may be the treatment of choice.

4. Intravenous verapamil should be used cautiously or avoided in patients with severe hypotension, poor left ventricular function or known conduction tissue disease.

REFERENCES

Bar FW, Brugada P, Dassen WRM:  Differential diagnosis of tachycardia with narrow QRS complex (shorter than 0.12 second).  Am J Cardiol 54:555, 1984.

Josephson ME, Kastor JA:  Supraventricular tachycardia:  Mechanisms and management.  Ann Intern Med 87:346, 1977.

Mauritson DR, Winniford MD, Walker WS:  Oral verapamil for paroxysmal supraventricular tachycardia.  Ann Intern Med 96:409, 1982.

Sung RJ, Elser B, McAllister RG Jr:  Intravenous verapamil for termination of reentrant supraventricular tachycardias: Intracardiac studies correlated with plasma verapamil concentrations.  Ann Intern Med 93:682, 1980.

## CASE 32: TACHYCARDIA AND SUDDEN COLLAPSE IN A YOUNG MAN

HISTORY

A 21-year-old male college student has enjoyed excellent health until he suddenly collapses while playing golf. Friends note that he transiently loses consciousness, and while paramedics are summoned, he awakens spontaneously but is lethargic, diaphoretic and ashen. The paramedics find shallow respirations, a blood pressure of 70 and palpable, and a heart rate in excess of 280 beats/minute and irregular. Cardiac monitoring shows a wide QRS complex. The patient is intubated and transported to the emergency room.

EXAMINATION

Physical examination shows a lethargic but responsive, well-nourished male with a blood pressure of 90/50, heart rate of 240 (irregular), and spontaneous respirations at 24. The lungs are clear; cardiac examination shows mild jugular venous distension.

ADDITIONAL DATA

Chest x-ray and electrolytes are normal.

CLUE FROM THE ECG

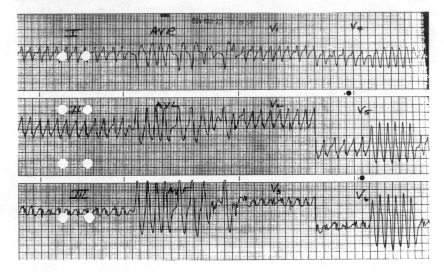

QUESTIONS

1. What is the diagnosis of this arrhythmia?
2. What is the significance of this arrhythmia?
3. What treatment should be administered?
4. What does the postconversion ECG show?
5. Should this patient be referred for electrophysiologic studies?

ANSWERS

1. Wolff-Parkinson-White syndrome (WPW). This is a preexcitation phenomenon secondary to atrioventricular (AV) transmission over a Kent bundle. ECG localization of the bypass fiber over the left AV groove is suggested by the presence of an initial negative deflection (delta wave = initial 200 msec in leads I and AVL). Two major dysrhythmic complications can occur with WPW: reentry tachycardia, via the accessory pathway, and atrial fibrillation. This patient demonstrates atrial fibrillation with a very rapid ventricular response, implying AV conduction via an accessory pathway.

2. This is a recognized medical emergency because of the high risk of this rhythm degenerating into ventricular fibrillation.

3. When life-threatening atrial fibrillation occurs, urgent therapy is required, and direct current cardioversion is recommended. When the blood pressure is adequate and tissue perfusion is maintained, drug therapy with intravenous procainamide (loading dose up to 1.0 g at a rate not to exceed 50 mg/minute) is an alternative choice.

4. The ECG shows a short PR interval and a delta wave (slurring of the upstroke of the QRS) characteristic of the Wolff-Parkinson-White syndrome:

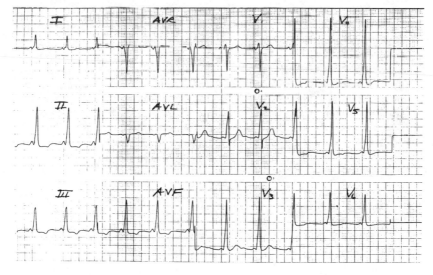

5. Electrophysiologic study is indicated in this patient with antegrade conduction via the accessory pathway resulting in a life-threatening arrhythmia.

## PEARLS

1. Patients with WPW syndrome have an increased incidence of atrial fibrillation, the mechanism of which is yet to be clarified.
2. The refractory period of the bypass tract is usually short and results in a very rapid ventricular response in atrial fibrillation.
3. Drugs that prolong the refractory period of the bypass tract, such as procainamide or quinidine, will slow the rate in atrial fibrillation with antegrade conduction.
4. Patients with atrial fibrillation, especially if symptomatic on drug therapy, are often candidates for surgical ablation of the bypass tract.
5. Although Kent bypass fibers may be located anywhere around the circumference of the right and left AV annuli, the majority are found in the left AV groove.

## PITFALLS

1. Digoxin and verapamil can potentially worsen the tachycardia in atrial fibrillation in the WPW syndrome; these drugs are contraindicated in this setting.
2. Beta blocker therapy, although effective in blocking enhanced sympathetic tone, does not lengthen  the effective refractory period of the bypass tract.  For this reason, propranolol as a single agent would be minimally effective in treating this patient's tachycardia.
3. Drug therapy in patients with WPW syndrome and palpitations should not be started until the exact nature of the arrhythmia is identified.

## REFERENCES

Dreifus LS, Haiat R, Watanabe Y:  Ventricular fibrillation:  A possible mechanism of sudden death in patients with Wolff-Parkinson-White syndrome.  Circulation 43:520, 1971.
Gallagher JJ, Pritchett E, Sealy WC, et al:  The preexcitation syndromes. Prog Cardiovasc Dis 20:285, 1978.

Gallagher JJ, Svenson RH, Casell JH, et al: Catheter technique for closed chest ablation of the atrioventricular conduction system. N Engl J Med 306:194, 1982.

Sellers TD, Bashore TM, Gallagher JJ: Digitalis in the pre-excitation syndrome: Analysis during atrial fibrillation. Circulation 56:260, 1977.

Wellens HJJ, Bar FW, Dassen WRM, et al: Effect of drugs in the Wolff-Parkinson-White syndrome: Importance of initial length of effective refractory period of the accessory pathway. Am J Cardiol 46:665, 1980.

Wellens HJJ, Bar FWHM, Lie KI: The value of the electrocardiogram in the difforontial diagnosis of a tachycardia with a widened QRS complex. Am J Med 64:27, 1978.

Wellens HJJ, Durrer D: Effect of digitalis on atrioventricular conduction and circus movement tachycardia in patients with Wolff-Parkinson-White syndrome. Circulation 47:1229, 1973.

## CASE 33: ABNORMAL ECG ON ROUTINE EXAM

HISTORY

A 35-year-old lawyer is told that his ECG obtained as part of a life insurance examination shows evidence of a prior heart attack. He denies any past symptoms such as chest discomfort or shortness of breath and has not seen a physician for any reason in the past 5 years. He has no history of palpitations, lightheadedness or syncope, and he plays singles tennis 3-4 times/week. He cannot recall ever having a previous ECG.

EXAMINATION

Physical examination shows a blood pressure of 124/76 and a heart rate of 82 and regular. The jugular venous pulsations, carotid pulse and remainder of the cardiac examination are within normal limits.

ADDITIONAL DATA

The chest x-ray shows a normal cardiac silhouette.

The ECG is shown below:

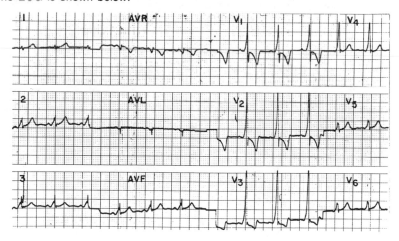

QUESTIONS

1. How would you interpret this ECG?
2. What further evaluation is warranted?
3. What recommendations would you give this patient?
4. What is the significance of atrial fibrillation in this syndrome?
5. What is this patient's prognosis?

ANSWERS

1. The ECG demonstrates the triad of: (1) short PR interval, (2) widened QRS complex, and (3) slurring of the upstroke of the QRS (delta wave) characteristic of the Wolff-Parkinson-White (WPW) syndrome. Q waves suggesting previous myocardial infarction are common in the WPW syndrome.

2. This patient has a normal history, examination and chest x-ray, and it is unlikely that further evaluation would uncover any underlying structural heart disease. In the absence of symptoms suggesting tachyarrhythmias, no further evaluation seems necessary. An echocardiogram could be done to exclude occult structural heart disease.

3. The patient should be informed that tachyarrhythmias can occur, and he should probably be taught the Valsalva maneuver to perform in the event of sustained palpitations.

4. Up to 20-25% of patients with WPW syndrome have atrial fibrillation; a subset of these will conduct antegrade along the anomalous atrioventricular connection. Heart rates may approach 300 beats/minute and deteriorate into ventricular fibrillation and sudden cardiac death.

5. This patient's prognosis is excellent. There is no convincing evidence that WPW syndrome patients without tachyarrhythmias have a higher expected mortality than patients with normal ECG's.

PEARLS

1. The WPW syndrome is seen in approximately 0.15% of the healthy population.

2. The WPW syndrome is due to conduction via anomalous pathways termed bundles of Kent; the widened QRS complex results from the fusion of ventricular activation occurring down the anomalous and normal conducting pathways.

3. The most common tachyarrhythmia in the preexcitation syndrome is reentrant supraventricular tachycardia (SVT) due to antegrade conduction down the normal His-Purkinje system with retrograde (ventriculoatrial) conduction along the anomalous pathway. The QRS complex of the WPW syndrome characteristically narrows during this type of SVT due to the loss of antegrade conduction down the bypass tract.

4. Delta waves may be seen intermittently. Some evidence suggests that this is associated with slower ventricular response rates in the event of atrial fibrillation.
5. Approximately 5% of patients with SVT have preexcitation; conversely, 50% of patients with preexcitation have a history of tachyarrhythmias.

PITFALLS

1. Patients with atrial fibrillation and antegrade conduction along anomalous pathways will have a wide QRS tachycardia that may resemble ventricular tachycardia.
2. Prompt cardioversion is recommended in patients with WPW syndrome and atrial fibrillation who have antegrade conduction with ventricular rates faster than 200-220/minute, because of the risk of ventricular fibrillation and death.
3. Patients with WPW syndrome have up to a 90% incidence of false positive ST segment changes during stress electrocardiography.

REFERENCES

Bardy GH, Packer DL, German LD, et al: Preexcited reciprocating tachycardia in patients with Wolff-Parkinson-White syndrome: Incidence and mechanisms. Circulation 70:377, 1984.

Gallagher JJ, Pritchett ELC, Sealy WC, et al: The preexcitation syndromes. Prog Cardiovasc Dis 20:285, 1978.

German LD, Gallagher JJ: Functional properties of accessory atrioventricular pathways in Wolff-Parkinson-White syndrome. Am J Med 76:1079, 1984.

Klein GJ, Bashore TM, Sellers TD, et al: Ventricular fibrillation in the Wolff-Parkinson-White syndrome. N Engl J Med 301:1080, 1979.

Klein GJ, Gulamhusein SS: Intermittent preexcitation in the Wolff-Parkinson-White syndrome. Am J Cardiol 52:292, 1983.

Richardson JM: Ventricular preexcitation: Practical considerations. Arch Intern Med 143:760, 1983.

Webb CR, Horowitz LN: Preexcitation syndromes: Principles and management. Cardiovasc Med 11:873, 1984.

## CASE 34: INTERMITTENT CHEST POUNDING AND LIGHTHEADEDNESS

HISTORY

A 64-year-old woman presents with a chief complaint of palpitations, weakness and near syncope. There is no history of prior cardiac disease. She has enjoyed excellent health until 1 year ago when transient (3-5 minute) episodes of a rapid pounding and irregular heartbeat were noted. These have occurred with sudden onset and have been associated with lightheadedness and near syncope. She has no risk factors for coronary artery disease.

EXAMINATION

Blood pressure is 150/96; heart rate is 56. The lung fields are clear, and the cardiovascular examination is normal except for an S4 gallop.

ADDITIONAL DATA

The ECG shows sinus bradycardia with minor NS-ST and T abnormalities and left ventricular hypertrophy. The chest x-ray shows a mildly tortuous aorta and no evidence of congestive heart failure.

Representative rhythm strips are shown below:

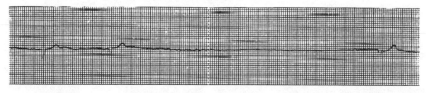

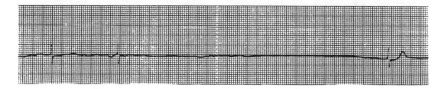

QUESTIONS

1. What is the diagnosis?
2. What is the mechanism of syncope in this syndrome?
3. What rhythm is likely to correlate with the patient's symptom of palpitations?
4. What is the best method of confirming this diagnosis?
5. Do these patients usually have underlying organic heart disease?
6. What is the optimal therapy for this syndrome?

ANSWERS

1. Sick sinus syndrome, also referred to as the "tachy-brady" syndrome.
2. Cardiac asystole and profound bradycardia are the most common causes of syncope or dizzy spells in this syndrome. In a smaller percentage of cases, symptoms may be the result of tachycardia.
3. The palpitations correlate with the tachycardia, which in the "tachy-brady" syndrome is most often atrial fibrillation, flutter or atrial tachycardia.
4. Ambulatory monitoring will confirm the diagnosis in the vast majority of cases. It is important to document that abnormal rhythms correlate with symptoms. Electrophysiologic studies can detect abnormalities of sinus node function in many patients; however, such evaluations sometimes reveal normal sinus node function in patients with symptomatic sinus node dysfunction during ambulatory ECG monitoring. In most cases, electrophysiologic studies are not necessary for diagnosis or management.
5. Some form of organic heart disease is present in more than 70% of the cases, with coronary artery disease, valvular heart disease, cardiomyopathy or hypertensive heart disease being common etiologies.
6. Once symptomatic bradycardia is confirmed by Holter monitoring, optimal therapy includes insertion of a permanent pacer. Treatment of the tachycardia can exacerbate bradycardia and therefore must be delayed (or used very cautiously, in borderline cases) until pacemaker insertion has been accomplished. Successful pacing generally relieves symptoms.

PEARLS

1. Nearly 75% of all pacemaker use in this country may be attributed to sick sinus syndrome.
2. Continuous ECG monitoring which documents a pause greater than 3-4 seconds in symptomatic patients will fulfill criteria for insertion of a permanent pacemaker.
3. Sudden death from sick sinus syndrome is rare.
4. Dual-chamber pacing is preferable in selected cases; this preserves atrial activity and optimizes cardiac output.

PITFALLS

1. Asymptomatic bradycardias which are clinically insignificant do not warrant pacemaker insertion.
2. Young people and well-conditioned athletes may spontaneously show pauses (up to 2.5 seconds, usually during sleep) which may appear pathologic but are essentially normal.
3. Carotid sinus massage may precipitate a dramatic pause or asystole in sick sinus syndrome and should be avoided in this setting.
4. Electrophysiologic studies are rarely necessary in the diagnosis and treatment of patients with sick sinus syndrome. A normal sinus node recovery time during electrophysiologic testing does not exclude sick sinus syndrome.
5. Bradycardias may be drug induced. This should be thoroughly evaluated prior to pacemaker implantation.

REFERENCES

Lipsli J, Cohen L, Espinoza J, et al: Value of Holter monitoring in assessing cardiac arrhythmias in symptomatic patients. Am J Cardiol 37:102, 1976.
Lister JW, Gosseline AJ, Savage PS: Obscure syncope and the sick sinus syndrome. PACE 1:68, 1978.
Moss AJ, Doirs RJ: Brady-tachy syndrome. Prog Cardiovasc Dis 16:439, 1974.
Narula OS, Gann D, Samet P: Prognostic value of H-V intervals. In Narula OS (ed): His Bundle Electrocardiography and Clinical Electrophysiology. Philadelphia, FA Davis, 1975.

## CASE 35: DIZZINESS AFTER PACEMAKER PLACEMENT

HISTORY

A 66-year-old librarian complains of episodes of lightheadedness after the implantation of a pacemaker. She has had a 3-year history of paroxysmal supraventricular tachycardia. Two weeks ago she had a near-syncopal episode associated with sinus bradycardia at a rate of 30 with frequent pauses of 3 seconds, and a single-chamber (ventricular inhibited, or VVI) pacemaker was placed. The implantation was uncomplicated, and for 48 hours in the hospital the pacemaker demonstrated appropriate sensing and capturing at a backup rate of 75. Since pacemaker implantation, she has experienced several bouts of lightheadedness. (She has not counted her heartbeat during these recent episodes.) Her only medication is propranolol 40 mg 3 times daily to control the tachyarrhythmias.

EXAMINATION

Heart rate is 80 and regular; blood pressure is 140/80, with the patient in either the supine or the standing position. The neck veins show occasional prominent (cannon) waves. The carotid upstroke is normal, and there are no bruits. The lungs are clear, and the cardiac examination is normal, except for intermittent paradoxical splitting of the 2nd heart sound.

ADDITIONAL DATA

The chest x-ray shows proper position of the lead in the right ventricular apex.

CLUE FROM THE ECG

This rhythm strip was recorded while the patient was symptomatic; her blood pressure dropped to 90/60:

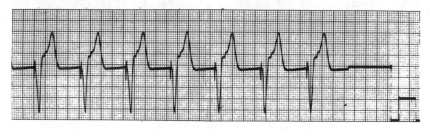

INTERPRETATION OF RHYTHM STRIP:   Ventricular pacing at a rate of 75; retrograde P waves follow each paced beat.

QUESTIONS

1.  What are the possible causes of the persistence of symptoms following pacemaker implantation?
2.  What is the mechanism of this clinical problem?
3.  What might the physical exam show during her symptoms with the rhythm strip above?
4.  What could be done to prevent further symptoms?

ANSWERS

1.  In this case, symptoms following pacemaker implantation are caused by altered hemodynamics from ventricular pacing, i.e., the pacemaker syndrome. Other causes include pacemaker failure, due to increasing threshold or lead dislodgement, and tachyarrhythmias.
2.  Mechanisms that have been postulated for the pacemaker syndrome include: loss of atrial contribution to ventricular filling; abnormal patterns of ventricular activation; atrial reflexes causing inappropriate vasodilatation; and functional valvular insufficiency.
3.  The patient's exam during pacing shows a drop in blood pressure and pulse pressure, regular cannon A waves, and paradoxical splitting of S2. Cannon waves are a sign of atrial contraction against the closed tricuspid valve; intermittent cannon waves suggest loss of atrioventricular (AV) synchrony, such as with heart block, ventricular tachycardia or ventricular pacing. Paradoxical splitting of the 2nd heart sound (splitting with expiration that narrows with inspiration) occurs when right ventricular activation precedes left ventricular (LV) activation, such as in left bundle branch block, right ventricular pacing, aortic stenosis or severe LV dysfunction.
4.  Therapy should be aimed at decreasing the periods of pacing, such as by lowering the backup rate to 50 and/or changing from the beta blocker to a drug less likely to cause sinus slowing. Rarely, changing to a dual-chamber pacemaker may be necessary to maintain AV synchrony.

PEARLS

1.  Ventriculoatrial conduction (with retrograde P waves) is present in the majority of patients who develop the pacemaker syndrome.
2.  Patients with carotid sinus hypersensitivity appear to be more likely to experience the pacemaker syndrome.

PITFALLS

1.  Although ventriculoatrial conduction may be a marker for patients who would develop the pacemaker syndrome, there is no reliable way to predict which patients will not tolerate single-chamber pacing.
2.  The atrial contribution to ventricular filling (and cardiac output) is particularly important for patients with noncompliant left ventricles

or severe LV dysfunction.

3. Chronic or recurrent atrial fibrillation remains a common contraindication for atrial sensing pacemakers that might otherwise be used to improve exercise capacity in patients needing artificial pacing.

## REFERENCES

Ausuber K, Furman S: The pacemaker syndrome. Ann Intern Med 103:420, 1985.

Nishimura RA, Gersh BJ, Holmes DR, et al: Outcome of dual-chamber pacing for the pacemaker syndrome. Mayo Clin Proc 58:452, 1983.

Nishimura RA, Gersh BJ, Vlietstra RE, et al: Hemodynamic and symptomatic consequences of ventricular pacing. PACE 5:903, 1982.

Perrins EJ, Morley CA, Chan SL, et al: Randomised controlled trial of physiological and ventricular pacing. Br Heart J 50:112, 1983.

Reiter MJ, Hindman MC: Hemodynamic effects of acute atrioventricular sequential pacing in patients with left ventricular dysfunction. Am J Cardiol 49:687, 1982.

## CASE 36: CHRONIC LUNG DISEASE AND IRREGULAR RHYTHM

HISTORY

A 62-year-old man is admitted to the intensive care unit (ICU) with severe dyspnea, cyanosis, fever and confusion. He has had a chronic, productive cough, a 60-pack-year history of smoking, and progressive edema with orthopnea. There is no prior history of heart disease. While he is in the ICU, rapid deterioration occurs despite vigorous bronchodilators and steroids, and intubation for ventilatory support is required. Cardiology consultation is requested because of a rapid, irregular rhythm.

EXAMINATION

Physical examination shows an elderly man with a blood pressure of 110/80 and heart rate of 140 with an irregular rhythm. The chest exam shows an increase in anterior-posterior diameter, hyperresonance to percussion, and generalized decreased breath sounds with wheezing and markedly prolonged expiration. The cardiac exam shows distant heart tones and a jugular venous pulse of 10 cm $H_2O$. Peripheral edema and hepatomegaly are noted.

CLUE FROM THE ECG

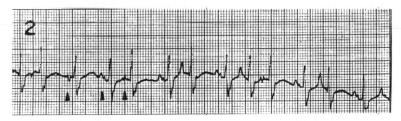

QUESTIONS

1.  What is this rapid, irregular heart rhythm?
2.  Why is this rhythm associated with a poor prognosis?
3.  What pharmacologic agents may provoke or worsen this condition?
4.  How do you treat this rhythm?

ANSWERS

1. Multifocal atrial tachycardia (MAT). This is an ectopic atrial arrhythmia with a rate exceeding 100 beats/minute with recognizable "P" waves from at least 3 distinct foci and with variable P-P, R-R and P-R intervals. It is a chaotic rhythm often confused with atrial fibrillation and may be due to enhanced atrial automaticity or "triggered activity."

2. Although the rhythm itself is not usually a direct cause of death, it is associated with a 50% mortality rate, because it occurs in the setting of severe pulmonary disease with acute or chronic respiratory failure.

3. Adrenergic bronchodilators, theophylline derivatives, vasopressors, inotropic agents and digoxin, especially at toxic levels, may facilitate the development of MAT. However, careful use of these agents may well play a role in reversing the underlying condition.

4. The treatment of MAT is based primarily on treating the underlying disorder and the accompanying metabolic abnormalities. Avoidance or correction of drug toxicities is important. Generally, drug therapy for the tachycardia itself is not necessary; when needed, the most useful drug is the calcium channel blocker verapamil.

PEARLS

1. MAT commonly resolves spontaneously when the underlying condition is treated.

2. The presence of cor pulmonale is particularly likely to predispose to the development of MAT.

3. The calcium channel-blocking agent verapamil has been shown to decrease the heart rate in MAT. In approximately 1/3 of patients it converts the rhythm to normal sinus. The usual initial dose is 5-10 mg intravenously.

PITFALLS

1. Because MAT is grossly similar to atrial fibrillation, digitalis is often tried as therapy. This is uniformly ineffective and may result in digitalis toxicity.

2. There may not be a consistent relationship between the severity of the underlying illness, i.e., respiratory failure, and the rhythm

disturbance.
3. The usual major antiarrhythmic agents (e.g., procainamide, quinidine, lidocaine) are not effective in controlling this dysrhythmia. Cardioversion is similarly ineffective for MAT.

## REFERENCES

Bisset GS, Seigel SF, Guam WE, et al:   Chaotic atrial tachycardia in childhood.   Am Heart J 101:268, 1981.

Chung EK:   Appraisal of multifocal atrial tachycardia.   Br Heart J 33:500, 1971.

Hagard PB, Burnett CR:   Treatment of multifocal atrial tachycardia with metoprolol.   Crit Care Med 15:20, 1987.

Levine JH, Michael JR, Guarnieri T:   Treatment of multifocal atrial tachycardia with verapamil.   N Engl J Med 312:21, 1985.

Levine JH, Michael JR, Guarnieri T:   Multifocal atrial tachycardia:   A toxic effect of theophylline.   Lancet 1:12, 1985.

Lipson MJ, Naimi S:   Multifocal atrial tachycardia (chaotic atrial tachycardia):   Clinical associations and significance.   Circulation 42:397, 1970.

Wang K, Goldfarb BL, Gobel FL, et al:   Multifocal atrial tachycardia:   A clinical analysis in 41 cases.   Arch Intern Med 137:161, 1977.

## CASE 37: SEVERE HYPERTENSION AND PAPILLEDEMA

HISTORY

A 43-year-old construction worker is referred by his ophthalmologist to the emergency room when his funduscopic examination shows papilledema. His blood pressure in the office is 240/140. The patient has had hypertension for over 10 years, treated with hydrochlorothiazide and prazosin; however, because he has felt well recently, he stopped his medications 2 weeks ago. Several days ago he noted frontal headaches and blurring of his vision, and for this reason saw his eye doctor. He has not had chest pain, shortness of breath, weakness or edema. There is no history of heart or kidney disease.

EXAMINATION

The patient is alert and in no distress. Blood pressure is 230/130; heart rate is 90 and regular. His eye grounds show blurred disk margins, arteriolar narrowing and several hemorrhages. The neck is supple; the lungs are clear without rales. The left ventricular impulse is slightly enlarged with a palpable presystolic impulse. There is an S4 gallop but no S3 or murmur. A neurologic exam shows normal mental status, gait and coordination.

ADDITIONAL DATA

The ECG shows left ventricular hypertrophy with strain. The chest x-ray shows mild cardiomegaly. Creatinine is 1.8 mg/dl.

CLUE FROM THE HISTORY AND EXAMINATION

The presence of papilledema in the setting of severe hypertension is indicative of early cerebral edema, which constitutes a hypertensive emergency.

QUESTIONS

1. What is the pathogenesis of hypertensive crisis?
2. What accelerated end-organ damage can be associated with severe hypertension?
3. Are diuretics appropriate therapy at this time?
4. How would you treat this patient?
5. To what levels should his blood pressure be reduced acutely?

ANSWERS

1. High blood pressure levels are associated with structural changes in renal and other arterioles. In addition, there is increased vascular reactivity, the release of vasoactive substances, and platelet aggregation with thrombosis and ischemia.
2. Hypertensive emergencies are accompanied by intracranial hemorrhage, hypertensive encephalopathy, acute pulmonary edema, aortic dissection, unstable angina or acute renal failure. Hypertensive urgencies are associated with minimal end-organ damage, milder funduscopic changes, or uncontrolled hypertension in the perioperative period.
3. No. Accelerated hypertension generally proceeds over several days and involves renal arteriolar constriction and diuresis. These patients are thus volume depleted, and further diuresis may cause clinical deterioration.
4. Prompt hospitalization and treatment with potent antihypertensives aimed at lowering the blood pressure within 1-2 hours are indicated. Oral clonidine, sublingual nifedipine, intravenous beta blockers, and vasodilators such as nitroprusside or hydralazine have all been used effectively.
5. These patients have compromised autoregulation of blood flow to the brain and other organs. They do not tolerate sudden lowering of blood pressure to normal levels. Initial therapy should be directed at maintaining diastolic blood pressure in the 100-110 range.

PEARLS

1. The duration of hypertension and the rate of the acceleration of the blood pressure are important determinants of end-organ damage; the absolute level of the blood pressure itself correlates poorly with the need for immediate intervention.
2. Angiotensin-converting enzyme inhibitors such as captopril or enalapril are particularly effective in the severe hypertension accompanying the renal crisis of scleroderma.
3. Pheochromocytoma should be suspected when malignant hypertension is sudden, intermittent and associated with headaches, excessive sweating or palpitations.

PITFALLS

1. The presence of severe hypertension with papilledema is associated with a 50% mortality over the next 5 years.
2. The abrupt withdrawal of moderate to high doses of clonidine may precipitate an acute hypertensive crisis.
3. In patients with cerebrovascular disease, rapid lowering of the blood pressure to "normal" levels may produce signs or symptoms of cerebral hypoperfusion with a loss of consciousness, transient ischemic attack or seizure.

REFERENCES

Anderson RJ, Hart GR, Crumpler CP, et al:  Oral clonidine loading in hypertensive urgencies.  JAMA 246:848, 1981.

Anderson RJ, Reed WG:  Current concepts in treatment of hypertensive urgencies.  Am Heart J 111:211, 1986.

Ferguson RK, Vlasses PH:  Hypertensive emergencies and urgencies.  JAMA 255:1607, 1986.

Houston M:  Hypertensive emergencies and urgencies:  Pathophysiology and clinical aspects.  Am Heart J 111:205, 1986.

Reed WG, Anderson RJ:  Effects of rapid blood pressure reduction on cerebral blood flow.  Am Heart J 111:226, 1986.

Vidt DG:  Current concepts in treatment of hypertensive emergencies.  Am Heart J 111:220, 1986.

## CASE 38: HYPERCHOLESTEROLEMIA

HISTORY

A 19-year-old college freshman is advised to have his cholesterol checked after his father suffers an acute myocardial infarction at age 43. He is of normal body weight, is active in sports at school, and has no history of diabetes or heart disease. Fasting triglyceride level is 105 mg/dl (normal less than 135); total cholesterol level is 320 mg/dl (greater than 95th percentile for age); high-density lipoprotein cholesterol (HDL-C) is 45 mg/dl (50th percentile). His father's cholesterol is 360 mg/dl (greater than 95th percentile).

EXAMINATION

There is a faint corneal arcus and nodular swelling and thickening of the Achilles tendons bilaterally; the remainder of the examination is normal.

CLUE FROM THE HISTORY AND EXAMINATION

This young man has severe hypercholesterolemia and tendinous xanthomas. The level of low-density lipoprotein cholesterol (LDL-C) can be estimated from the equation:

$$LDL\text{-}C = (\text{Total cholesterol}) - (\text{HDL-C}) - (\text{Triglycerides}/5)$$

In this patient, LDL-C = 244 mg/dl (95th percentile for age is 150).

QUESTIONS

1. What is the likely diagnosis of this man's hyperlipidemia?
2. What is the abnormality on a molecular/genetic level?
3. What further tests would you recommend?
4. What dietary advice will you give him?
5. How would you treat him in addition to diet?

ANSWERS

1. The pattern of increased cholesterol with normal triglycerides and HDL-C is due to elevation of the cholesterol-rich LDL particle with normal levels of the triglyceride-rich VLDL particle (type IIA hyperlipoproteinemia). The combination of high LDL-C, the familial tendency for hypercholesterolemia, and tendinous xanthomas suggests the diagnosis of familial hypercholesterolemia.

2. Familial hypercholesterolemia is due to abnormalities in one or both genes coding for the LDL receptors (gene frequency 1/500). In the heterozygous state, there are 50% of the normal number of LDL receptors, and cholesterol levels are in the 300-400 range.

3. Secondary causes of hypercholesterolemia, such as hypothyroidism and nephrotic syndrome, should be sought when elevated cholesterol levels are found. In addition, a baseline ECG should be obtained because of the development of coronary artery disease early in this disorder.

4. The diet should be low in saturated fats (red meat, dairy products, fats generally solid at room temperature) with substitution of vegetable oils high in polyunsaturated fats (e.g., safflower and sunflower oils). In severe cases dietary cholesterol should be limited to 100-200 mg/day.

5. The 2 types of pharmacologic agents most useful for lowering cholesterol are nicotinic acid (niacin) and the bile acid-binding resins (cholestyramine and colestipol). Recent studies show that specific inhibitors of the enzyme hepatic hydroxymethylglutaryl coenzyme A reductase, such as lovastatin, block the rate-limiting step in cholesterol synthesis and lower cholesterol levels an average of 25-40%.

PEARLS

1. Tendinous xanthomas are characteristic of familial hypercholesterol-emia and involve the Achilles tendons in over 75% of affected individuals.

2. Eighty-five percent of males and nearly 60% of females with familial hypercholesterolemia who remain untreated will have a myocardial infarction by the age of 60.

3. Diabetes mellitus and obesity are commonly seen in lipid disorders

associated with hypertriglyceridemia but not in those associated with isolated hypercholesterolemia.

4. A cholesterol level of 300 mg/dl results in a 4-fold greater risk of coronary artery disease than does a level of 200 mg/dl.
5. The majority of patients with hypercholesterolemia have polygenic hypercholesterolemia with levels in the range of 250-300 mg/dl.
6. Familial combined hyperlipidemia, inherited in an autosomal dominant fashion, is a relatively common disorder that can present as elevated triglycerides, elevated cholesterol, or both.
7. The HDL particle is thought to be protective; a low level of HDL-C has been shown in some studies to be an independent risk factor for atherosclerotic coronary artery disease.
8. Eruptive xanthomas over the trunk are characteristic of severe elevations of triglycerides due to high levels of chylomicrons in the blood, as seen in lipoprotein lipase deficiency.
9. One egg yolk contains approximately 250 mg of cholesterol.

PITFALLS

1. Treatment of hypercholesterolemia with bile acid-binding resins can cause triglycerides to increase significantly.
2. Nearly all drugs that lower cholesterol are associated with significant side effects or potential for toxicity that frequently limit their use.
3. Levels of the apolipoproteins A and B--specific surface proteins of the HDL and LDL particles, respectively--may prove to be better predictors of atherosclerotic disease than the HDL and LDL cholesterol levels.

REFERENCES

Anderson KM, Castelli WP, Levy D: Cholesterol and mortality: 30 years of follow-up from the Framingham study. JAMA 257:2176, 1987.
Goldstein JL, Brown MS: Genetics and cardiovascular disease. In Braunwald E (ed): Heart Disease: A Textbook of Cardiovascular Medicine. Philadelphia, WB Saunders, 1984.
Kottke BA: Hyperlipoproteinemia: The case for individualized care. Consultant 26:160, 1986.
Kottke BA, Zinsmeister AR, Holmes DR Jr, et al: Apolipoproteins and coronary artery disease. Mayo Clin Proc 61:313, 1986.

Levy RI, Feinleib M: Risk factors for coronary artery disease and their management. In Braunwald E (ed): Heart Disease: A Textbook of Cardiovascular Medicine. Philadelphia, WB Saunders, 1984.

Lipid Research Clinics Program: The Lipid Research Clinics coronary primary prevention trial results: I. Reduction in incidence of coronary heart disease. JAMA 251:351, 1984.

Lipid Research Clinics Program: The Lipid Research Clinics coronary primary prevention trial results: II. The relationship of reduction in incidence of coronary heart disease to cholesterol lowering. JAMA 251:365, 1984.

## CASE 39: YOUNG WOMAN WITH PROGRESSIVE DYSPNEA

HISTORY

A 30-year-old previously healthy housewife has noticed a slow onset of shortness of breath and a decrease in exercise tolerance over the past 6 months. She complains now that she becomes winded when she carries groceries or attempts to walk up 2 flights of stairs. Her only medication is birth control pills, which she has been taking for 6 years. She does not smoke cigarettes.

EXAMINATION

Heart rate is 90 and regular; blood pressure is 110/68. She is thin but does not appear chronically ill. The jugular venous pressure is elevated to 12 cm $H_2O$ with prominent A and V waves. The carotid volume is slightly decreased with a normal upstroke; her lungs are clear. The left ventricular (LV) impulse is normal, but there is a left parasternal lift and a palpable 2nd heart sound in the 3rd left intercostal space. There is a faint holosystolic murmur at the lower left sternal border, which increases during inspiration, and a II/VI early diastolic murmur along the upper left sternal border.

ADDITIONAL DATA

The chest x-ray shows dilated left and right pulmonary arteries and peripheral "pruning"; the overall heart size is normal with decrease in the anterior "clear space" on the lateral projection.

The ECG shows right ventricular hypertrophy.

QUESTIONS

1. What is the most likely diagnosis?
2. What are the pathologic subgroups of this disorder?
3. What are the most common symptoms at time of presentation?
4. What treatment would you recommend?
5. What is this patient's prognosis?

ANSWERS

1.  Primary pulmonary hypertension (PPH). Diagnostic studies should be vigorously undertaken to exclude treatable causes of "secondary" pulmonary hypertension, including occult mitral stenosis, intracardiac shunts, cor triatriatum, pulmonary embolic disease and collagen vascular disease.
2.  Examination of lung biopsies has revealed 2 major pathologic subgroups: thromboembolic (possibly due to in situ thrombosis) and plexogenic (characterized by obstructive arterial plexiform lesions). Other histologic forms include veno-occlusive disease, primary arteritis and arterial medial hypertrophy.
3.  The most common symptoms in this disorder are exertional dyspnea, syncope, fatigue and chest pain that may be anginal in nature.
4.  The treatment of primary pulmonary hypertension is mainly supportive. Discontinuation of oral contraceptives is mandatory, because they have been implicated as a cause of the disorder. Oxygen is recommended for hypoxemia, and treatment for clinical right-sided congestive heart failure may be necessary. Most authors now recommend long-term oral anticoagulation, which has been shown to prolong survival in some studies. Although response to vasodilators may identify a subgroup with improved survival, there is little proof that long-term vasodilator therapy will prolong life in these patients. Heart-lung transplantation is being investigated in selected centers.
5.  Unfortunately, prognosis in this disorder is poor, with average survival of only 20% at 5 years in most series.

PEARLS

1.  Primary pulmonary hypertension occurs predominantly in women.
2.  The mean age at diagnosis for this disorder is 34 years.
3.  The most common cause of pulmonary hypertension is "left-sided" lesions, including LV dysfunction, mitral stenosis and intracardiac shunts.
4.  Arterial desaturation, which occurs late in the disease, is due to right-to-left shunting through the foramen ovale or markedly impaired cardiac output.
5.  Raynaud's phenomenon is seen in 10-30% of patients with PPH.

6.  The diffusing capacity is the most likely pulmonary function test to be abnormal in the asymptomatic period of the illness.

PITFALLS

1.  PPH is characterized by a long latent period; symptoms occur late in the disorder and are usually associated with a rapid progression.
2.  The mechanics of breathing, as measured by the FEV1 and forced vital capacity, may be normal or near normal despite markedly elevated pulmonary pressures.
3.  Pulmonary angiography may be particularly hazardous in patients with severe pulmonary hypertension and has been associated with fatal outcome.
4.  Vasodilators should be used with caution in PPH. These drugs may preferentially dilate the systemic resistance vessels and precipitously drop systemic blood pressure. In some cases they may cause sudden death.

REFERENCES

Bjornsson J, Edwards WD: Primary pulmonary hypertension: A histopathologic study of 80 cases. Mayo Clin Proc 60:16, 1985.
Fuster V, Steele PM, Edwards WD, et al: Primary pulmonary hypertension: Natural history and the importance of thrombosis. Circulation 70:580, 1984.
McGoon MD, Edwards WD: Primary pulmonary hypertension: Current status. Mod Concepts Cardiovasc Dis 54:29, 1985.
Rich S, Brundage BH, Levy PS: The effect of vasodilator therapy on the clinical outcome of patients with primary pulmonary hypertension. Circulation 71:1191, 1985.

## CASE 40: PREOPERATIVE CLEARANCE IN A PATIENT WITH ANGINA PECTORIS

HISTORY

A surgeon asks you to evaluate a 64-year-old plumber who is to undergo cholecystectomy following an episode of cholecystitis. The patient sustained an uncomplicated inferior wall myocardial infarction (MI) 3 years ago. Since that time he has been treated with propranolol and sublingual isosorbide for angina pectoris that occurs with moderate to heavy exertion. There is no history of a heart murmur or congestive heart failure (CHF).

EXAMINATION

Blood pressure is 140/80; heart rate is 78 and regular. There is no jugular venous distension, and the carotid pulsations are normal. The lungs are clear; there is a normal left ventricular (LV) impulse, an apical S4, and no heart murmur or 3rd heart sound.

ADDITIONAL DATA

The ECG shows an old inferior wall infarction, right bundle branch block and no premature atrial or ventricular contractions and is unchanged from a recent record. The chest x-ray is normal.

CLUE FROM THE HISTORY AND EXAMINATION

This patient has stable angina pectoris and is without a recent myocardial infarction. In addition, there is no evidence for CHF, valvular aortic stenosis or abnormal rhythm.

QUESTIONS

1. What is the patient's risk of having an infarction at the time of his cholecystectomy?
2. What factors have been shown to correlate with an increased risk in the perioperative period?
3. How should his antianginal medications be administered during this time?
4. Is a preoperative treadmill test indicated?
5. Should a Swan-Ganz catheter be inserted prophylactically?
6. Should a temporary pacemaker be inserted?

ANSWERS

1. Patients with chronic, stable angina have a 5% incidence of perioperative cardiac event (MI, CHF or cardiac death) following noncardiac surgery. Prior MI within 3 months is associated with a 30% risk of a life-threatening cardiac event; this risk decreases to 15% at 3 months after infarction and plateaus at 5% after 6 months. Therefore, whenever possible, it is strongly recommended to wait at least 6 months after MI before elective surgery is undertaken.

2. In a large series published by Goldman et al. (reference), multivariate analysis identified 9 risk factors for cardiac events following noncardiac surgery:
   a. Age > 70.
   b. MI in previous 6 months.
   c. S3 gallop or jugular venous distension.
   d. Important valvular aortic stenosis.
   e. Rhythm other than sinus or PAC's.
   f. Five PVC's/minute any time preoperatively.
   g. Poor general status (hypoxemia, azotemia, abnormal liver function tests).
   h. Emergency surgery.
   i. Intraperitoneal, intrathoracic or aortic surgery.

3. The patient's propranolol and isosorbide should be continued up to and including the morning of surgery. Several studies have documented the safety of continuing antianginal medication in this fashion. In addition, there is a potential risk of rebound ischemia if beta blockers or nitrates are withdrawn prior to surgery. Propranolol should be resumed as soon as the patient is able to take oral medications; it can be given intravenously if a prolonged period of fasting is anticipated.

4. There are no controlled studies that support the routine use of preoperative exercise stress testing in asymptomatic patients or patients with stable angina.

5. Balloon-directed right heart catheterization is considered in a patient with a history of CHF, recent infarction, significant valvular disease or depressed LV function (LV ejection fraction, 35-40%). This patient has none of the usual indications for right heart catheterization, preoperatively.

6. Pacing is not indicated in this patient. Patients with asymptomatic right or left bundle branch block (or right bundle branch block and left

axis deviation) have no increase in mortality with general anesthesia and surgery.

PEARLS

1. Up to 1/2 of all deaths complicating noncardiac surgery are due to cardiovascular causes, and the majority of these occur in patients with known cardiac disease.
2. Thirty to 40% of patients with CHF, as evidenced by rales and S3 gallop, will have a life-threatening or fatal cardiac event following noncardiac surgery.
3. The peak incidence of perioperative MI following surgery is on postoperative day 3.
4. Herniorrhaphy, transurethral resection of the prostate and operations performed with regional anesthesia confer minimal operative risk, even in patients with underlying heart disease.
5. New, sustained supraventricular tachycardia occurs in 10-15% of patients over the age of 60 undergoing thoracic operations.

PITFALLS

1. Approximately 50% of patients with perioperative MI's do not experience chest pain; diagnosis is made by routine ECG or during evaluation of postoperative CHF or ventricular ectopy.
2. Spinal anesthesia may result in hypotension due to vasodilation and is no safer than general anesthesia in patients with cardiac disease.
3. Initiating digitalis administration is not warranted in patients with compensated CHF; digitalis toxicity in the perioperative period may be precipitated by hypoxemia, hypokalemia or alkalosis.
4. Mortality for a perioperative MI is 20-30%, if it is a 1st MI, and as high as 50-70%, if it is a 2nd infarction.
5. Hypertension with diastolic blood pressure up to 100-110 mm Hg is not an independent risk factor; overly aggressive preoperative therapy, however, may induce hypovolemia and/or hypokalemia, which may be of significant risk.

REFERENCES

Carliner NH, Fisher ML, Plotnick GD, et al: Routine preoperative exercise testing in patients undergoing major noncardiac surgery. Am J Cardiol 56:51, 1985.

Goldman L: Supraventricular tachyarrhythmias in hospitalized adults after surgery. Chest 73:450, 1978.

Goldman L: Noncardiac surgery in patients receiving propranolol. Arch Intern Med 141:193, 1981.

Goldman L: Cardiac risks and complications of noncardiac surgery. Ann Surg 198:780, 1983.

Goldman L, Caldera DL, Nussbaum SR, et al: Multifactorial index of cardiac risk in noncardiac surgical procedures. N Engl J Med 297:845, 1977.

Goldman L, Caldera DL, Southwick FS, et al: Cardiac risk factors and complications in noncardiac surgery. Medicine 57:357, 1978.

Rose SD, Corman LC, Mason DT: Cardiac risk factors in patients undergoing noncardiac surgery. Med Clin North Am 63:1271, 1979.

Steen PA, Tinker JH, Tarhan S: Myocardial reinfarction after anesthesia and surgery. JAMA 239:2566, 1978.

## CASE 41: HEART FAILURE, NAUSEA AND RHYTHM CHANGE IN AN ELDERLY MAN

HISTORY

Two months ago, a 79-year-old hypertensive man presented with symptoms of dyspnea and edema and was noted to be in congestive heart failure. Treatment was initiated with digoxin 0.25 mg and furosemide 40 mg daily, and improvement followed. Two weeks ago, he presented with worsening dyspnea, fatigue and recurrence of edema. The heart rate was 100; pulse was irregular. After an ECG confirmed the presence of atrial fibrillation, treatment with quinidine gluconate was initiated, and furosemide was increased to 80 mg/day.

Now, the dyspnea has resolved, but he complains of a loss of appetite, nausea and vomiting.

EXAMINATION

Physical examination reveals a blood pressure of 130/80; heart rate is 90 and regular. Lungs are clear to auscultation and percussion. Cardiac examination shows no murmurs or gallops. The abdomen reveals mild generalized tenderness with guarding, and bowel sounds are present.

ADDITIONAL DATA

The ECG shows atrial fibrillation with a regular ventricular response. Electrolytes: blood urea nitrogen = 38 mg/dl; creatinine - 1.7 mg/dl; $K_i$ = 2.8 mEq/liter; and Na+ = 132 mEq/liter. Digoxin level = 3.2 ng/ml (reference range, 0.9-2.4 ng/ml).

QUESTIONS

1. What factors have contributed to the development of digitalis toxicity?
2. What rhythm disturbances are commonly seen with digitalis toxicity, and specifically, what manifestation of toxicity is encountered in this case?
3. What treatment is recommended?
4. What percentage of digoxin is metabolized daily with normal renal function, and how does renal impairment affect clearance?
5. Does digitalis toxicity occur predictably at a given digoxin level?

ANSWERS

1. The addition of quinidine will raise the circulating level of digoxin by decreasing the volume of distribution and reducing renal clearance. Other factors contributing to this syndrome are the presence of hypokalemia and renal insufficiency, as digoxin is excreted by the kidneys. Advanced age also predisposes to digitalis toxicity.

2. Ventricular premature complexes, especially ventricular bigeminy and 1st and 2nd degree atrioventricular (AV) block, are the most commonly encountered arrhythmias. In patients with atrial fibrillation who are taking digoxin and who develop a regular tachycardia or a slow ventricular rate, a diagnosis of digitalic toxicity is strongly suggested. On rare occasions, ventricular tachycardia or ventricular fibrillation can occur.

3. Treatment should be initiated promptly, with attention directed at correcting volume status and potassium level. The magnesium level should be checked and restored to normal. If significant ventricular ectopy occurs, lidocaine or phenytoin is indicated. If rapid junctional tachycardia results in a compromised hemodynamic status, phenytoin followed by procainamide and, perhaps, beta blockers can be used. For life-threatening digoxin toxicity, urgent administration of digitalis antibodies (glycoside-specific Fab fragments) should be undertaken.

4. Approximately 1/3 of the body's store of digoxin is eliminated daily if renal function is normal. When renal insufficiency is present, as with this patient, clearance is delayed. The hepatic contribution to daily elimination is 14%.

5. No. Since the effects of digoxin are in part dependent on the metabolic milieu, toxicity may be manifest at a normal digoxin level, if hypokalemia or hypomagnesemia is present, or with thyrotoxicosis, hypoxemia or alkalemia.

PEARLS

1. Arrhythmias from digitalis toxicity may take the form of almost any rhythm disturbance.

2. Think of digitalis toxicity when regular rhythms become irregular or when irregular rhythms become regular.

3. Digitalis toxicity is a clinical diagnosis; digitalis levels help to confirm this entity. An elevated serum level in the absence of

clinical toxicity should not be used to establish the diagnosis.
4. Serious or life-threatening overdoses of digoxin should be treated with glycoside-specific (Fab fragment) antibodies.

## PITFALLS

1. Routine determination of digitalis levels should be discouraged. Levels are most useful in confirming the clinical diagnosis of toxicity and in evaluating patient compliance with drug therapy.
2. Lack of recognition of digitalis toxicity is a common and potentially serious problem.
3. Hypokalemia will worsen the dysrhythmia induced by digitalis and must be treated. However, in massive digitalis overdose, release of intracellular potassium may result in severe hyperkalemia.
4. Advanced age is associated with a higher likelihood of digitalis toxicity because of the common problems of reduced renal, pulmonary and cardiac function, as well as the increased percentage of patients on multiple drugs.

## REFERENCES

Aronson JK, Grahave-Smith DG: Digoxin therapy: Textbooks, therapy and practice. Br J Clin Pharmacol 3:639, 1976.

Doerry W: Quinidine-digoxin interaction, pharmacokinetics underlying mechanisms and clinical implications. N Engl J Med 301:400, 1979.

Hager WD, Feuster P, Mayersohn M, et al: Digoxin-quinidine interaction: Pharmacokinetic evaluation. N Engl J Med 300:1238, 1979.

Moysey JO, Jugyaro NSU, Grundy EN, et al: Amiodarone increases plasma digoxin concentrations. Br Med J 282:372, 1984.

Shapiro W: Correlative studies of 7 digitalis levels and the arrhythmias of digitalis intoxication. Am J Cardiol 41:852, 1978.

## CASE 42: SYNCOPE

HISTORY

A 64-year-old housewife is brought to the emergency room after a syncopal episode in the market. She is now awake and alert and remembers only feeling suddenly lightheaded while pushing her shopping cart. According to her husband, who witnessed the event, she suddenly slumped to the floor and was unconscious for 5-10 seconds; there was no seizure activity or period of confusion after she awakened spontaneously. She does not remember any awareness of her heartbeat or chest discomfort. There is no history of seizures, orthostatic lightheadedness, heart murmur or angina. Approximately 2 years ago she had a similar episode without true loss of consciousness, for which she did not seek medical attention. She is otherwise very healthy, and her only medication is hydrochlorothiazide for hypertension.

EXAMINATION

An alert woman, oriented and in no distress. Blood pressure is 146/78; heart rate is 64 and regular with the patient supine. There is no change in blood pressure with standing. There are no carotid bruits. The cardiac and neurologic examinations are entirely normal. Carotid sinus massage causes slowing of the heart rate to 48 with an asymptomatic 1.8-second pause.

ADDITIONAL DATA

The ECG is normal. Hemoglobin is 13.6 g/dl. Electrolytes: blood urea nitrogen = 20 mg/dl; creatinine = 1.1 mg/dl; K+ = 3.3 mEq/liter; and Na+ = 136 mEq/liter.

CLUE FROM THE HISTORY AND EXAMINATION

The initial history and physical examination do not provide any significant clues to the cause of this syncopal episode.

QUESTIONS

1. What is the likely cause of this woman's syncope?
2. What further evaluation would you recommend?
3. What is her prognosis?
4. What is the likelihood that an electroencephalogram (EEG) or computerized axial tomography (CT) of the head will aid in the diagnosis?
5. How might electrophysiologic (EP) studies be useful in this patient with syncope?
6. How would you follow this patient?

## ANSWERS

1. The term that is currently used to describe syncope in which there is no diagnosis apparent after careful history, physical examination (including postural vital signs, neurologic examination, carotid sinus massage) and basic laboratory testing (screening blood work, ECG) is "syncope of unknown origin."

2. Holter monitoring and in-hospital cardiac monitoring remain useful tools in the diagnosis of syncope; either might be recommended in this patient.

3. Patients with syncope for which no specific cause can be identified ("syncope of unknown origin") are at relatively low risk, with a 1-year mortality of 1-5%; mortality is related to age and to the presence of serious underlying illness.

4. In several large studies of patients presenting to the emergency room or to medical clinics with the diagnosis of syncope, head CT and EEG rarely showed abnormalities associated with the cause of syncope in the absence of focal neurologic findings or history of seizures. Thus, most authors do not recommend these tests routinely.

5. The indications for EP studies in patients with syncope of unknown origin are not well defined, particularly in the absence of underlying heart disease. Fewer than 20% of women, such as this patient, without suspected structural heart disease will have supraventricular or ventricular tachyarrhythmias inducible in the EP laboratory that would explain the syncopal episode. Those with conduction system abnormalities responsible for syncope will generally have the diagnosis made from ambulatory monitoring and will not require EP studies for diagnosis.

6. The only follow-up that is necessary in the absence of further symptoms is routine clinical care. Symptoms referable to the cardiovascular system should be sought on subsequent visits, but no specific testing would be recommended without further indication.

## PEARLS

1. The cause of syncope, especially in the elderly, is often multifactorial, and a single diagnosis may not explain the syncopal episode.

2. Approximately 85% of the diagnoses of syncope (in cases for which a diagnosis is ultimately made) are made from the history, physical

examination and initial ECG; most of the remaining diagnoses are made by prolonged ECG monitoring.

3. Patients with the diagnosis of syncope of cardiac origin comprise approximately 10% of patients presenting to the emergency room and are at highest risk, with a 1-year mortality of 20-30%.

4. Psychogenic or vasovagal syncope comprises approximately 40-50% of cases evaluated in the emergency room.

PITFALLS

1. All prospective and retrospective studies on syncope differ in terms of entry criteria, mode of entry (emergency room versus hospital), inclusion of seizures, diagnostic evaluation, length of follow-up, etc. Thus, generalizations regarding the prevalence, prognosis and optimal evaluation of patients with syncope must be made cautiously.

2. Patients over the age of 70 with syncope of unknown origin or those with syncope due to central nervous system or metabolic cause comprise a heterogeneous group whose risk for recurrences or mortality cannot easily be defined.

REFERENCES

Day SC, Cook EF, Funkenstein H, et al:   Evaluation and outcome of emergency room patients with transient loss of consciousness.   Am J Med 73:15, 1982.

Eagle KA, Black HR, Cook EF, Goldman L:   Evaluation and prognostic classifications for patients with syncope.   Am J Med 79:455, 1985.

Kapoor WN, Karpf M, Maher Y, et al:   Syncope of unknown origin: The need for a more cost-effective approach to its diagnostic evaluation. JAMA 247:2687, 1982.

Kapoor WN, Karpf M, Wiland S, et al:   A prospective evaluation and follow-up of patients with syncope.   N Engl J Med 309:197, 1983.

Morady F, Shen E, Schwartz A, et al:   Long-term follow-up of patients with recurrent unexplained syncope evaluated by electrophysiologic testing.   J Am Coll Cardiol 2:1053, 1983.

Teichman SL, Felder SD, Matos JA, et al:   The value of electrophysiologic studies in syncope of undetermined origin:   Report of 150 cases.   Am Heart J 110:469, 1985.

## CASE 43: FEVER AND ABNORMAL HEART EXAM

HISTORY

You are asked to see a 58-year-old housewife who has been admitted for evaluation of a fever of 3 weeks duration. The patient denies prior rheumatic fever or history of any cardiac disease. She has noticed some dyspnea on exertion during the past 6 months and low-grade fevers beginning nearly a month ago. Review of systems elicits the history of an episode of transient right eye blindness lasting several minutes 2 months ago, for which she did not seek medical attention.

EXAMINATION

Heart rate is 92; blood pressure is 110/76; temperature is 38.3ºC. The patient is a thin female in no acute distress. Her skin reveals several splinter hemorrhages. Heart examination shows a regular rhythm. There is a left parasternal lift and palpable P2. S1 is prominent with a normal 2nd heart sound. There is an early diastolic sound followed by a low-pitched diastolic murmur at the apex.

ADDITIONAL DATA

Hemoglobin is 10.6 g/100 ml. The ECG shows sinus rhythm and left atrial abnormality. The chest x-ray shows mild pulmonary vascular redistribution.

CLUE FROM THE ECHOCARDIOGRAM

The 2-dimensional echocardiogram (parasternal long axis view) is shown below:

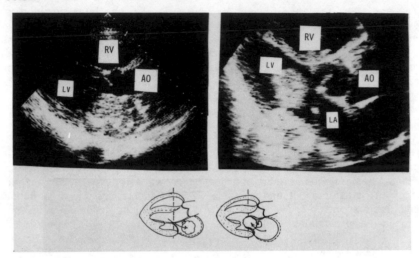

Figure A. AO = aorta; LA = left atrium; LV = left ventricle;
RV = right ventricle.

QUESTIONS

1. What diagnosis suggested by the echocardiogram is most compatible with the patient's history?
2. What other diagnoses should be considered from the history and examination?
3. What is the origin of the left atrial mass?
4. What therapy is indicated?
5. How should this patient be evaluated following definitive therapy?

ANSWERS

1. The echocardiogram demonstrates a pedunculated left atrial mass that extends through the mitral valve and is most likely a left atrial myxoma.
2. The examination, ECG and chest x-ray suggest pulmonary hypertension due to rheumatic mitral stenosis. Another important consideration in a patient with fever, murmurs and evidence of embolic phenomena is the diagnosis of infective endocarditis. Other diagnoses to be investigated in this patient include systemic lupus erythematosus (and other vasculitides) and occult malignancy.
3. Left atrial myxomas histologically resemble pluripotential mesenchymal cells; recent studies have demonstrated high levels of factor VIII-related antigen, suggesting an endothelial (or endocardial) origin of the benign neoplasm. The tumor does not appear to arise from thrombus, as was previously postulated.
4. Resection is curative in the majority of cases and should be undertaken even in asymptomatic patients with left atrial myxomas.
5. Long-term follow-up should include serial echocardiograms because of the 4-5% recurrence rate in patients who have had myxomas resected.

PEARLS

1. Atrial myxoma is the most common intracavitary cardiac tumor, accounting for 40% of all benign cardiac tumors.
2. Myxomas generally present in the 5th and 6th decade and demonstrate a 3:1 female:male predominance.
3. Three-fourths of myxomas occur in the left atrium and are most commonly attached to the interatrial septum near the fossa ovalis.
4. The murmurs due to atrial myxomas may dramatically change with the position of the patient; similarly, patients may describe improvement in their symptoms when they lie down (due to posterior displacement of the tumor away from the mitral valve orifice).
5. Dyspnea on exertion is the most common presenting symptom and is of more recent onset and more rapidly progressive than is the dyspnea due to rheumatic mitral stenosis.
6. Embolic phenomena are the initial presenting symptoms in nearly 25% of patients with left atrial myxoma.

PITFALLS

1. Because of the protean manifestations and subtle symptoms, the diagnosis of atrial myxoma in some patients may be delayed for years.
2. The early diastolic sound or "tumor plop" followed by the diastolic rumbling murmur mimics the opening snap and murmur of a stenotic mitral valve and may strongly suggest the diagnosis of rheumatic heart disease.
3. The vast majority of left atrial tumors are benign myxomas, whereas the majority of right atrial tumors are malignant; when right atrial myxoma is suspected, studies should be undertaken to exclude renal cell carcinoma and other malignancies that can invade the vena cava and right atrium.
4. Cardiac catheterization may not be necessary, as the anatomic characteristics are usually well delineated by the noninvasive techniques of 2-dimensional echocardiography and magnetic resonance imaging. Forward angiography with a pulmonary artery contrast injection may be performed, but transseptal catheterization is thought to be contraindicated.

REFERENCES

Bloor CM, O'Rourke RA: Cardiac tumors: Clinical presentations and pathologic correlations. Curr Probl Cardiol 9:3, 1984.
Bulkley BH, Hutchins GM: Atrial myxomas: A fifty-year review. Am Heart J 97:639, 1979.
Fisher J: Cardiac myxoma. Cardiovasc Rev Rep 4:1195, 1983.

## CASE 44:  MULTIPLE ADMISSIONS FOR PULMONARY EDEMA

HISTORY

A 64-year-old gas station owner presents with acute pulmonary edema. The patient has had 3 hospitalizations for heart failure in the past year and has been on digitalis and furosemide for 1 year. He has a history of a large anterior myocardial infarction which occurred 3 years ago. His risk factors include hypertension, smoking and hypercholesterolemia. He has had frequent ventricular ectopic beats since his infarction.

EXAMINATION

On initial physical examination the blood pressure is 150/90, heart rate is 130, and respiratory rate is 28. The patient is an acutely ill, anxious and overweight male in respiratory distress. The apical impulse is enlarged and felt in the 6th intercostal space in the anterior axillary line. There is a regular rhythm with an occasional ectopic beat. A gallop is present, and a soft systolic murmur at the apex is noted. There is no hepatomegaly or peripheral edema. There are diffuse rales.

ADDITIONAL DATA

The chest x-ray shows pulmonary edema and cardiomegaly.

CLUE FROM THE ECG's

ECG after his heart attack 3 years ago:

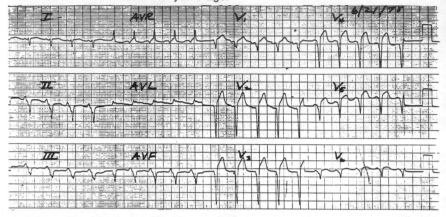

ECG on this admission:

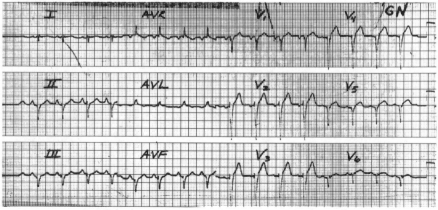

INTERPRETATION OF ECG's: The tracings show evidence of a large anterolateral myocardial infarction with ST segment elevation, sinus tachycardia, and left atrial abnormality. The axis is superior and rightward. There is no significant change between the 2 tracings.

HOSPITAL COURSE

The patient is treated with oxygen, furosemide and morphine sulfate and improves quickly.    Serial creatine kinase determinations are normal. There are no serial ECG changes.

QUESTIONS

1.  What is the underlying etiology of this man's left-sided congestive heart failure?
2.  What noninvasive tests would be helpful in confirming the diagnosis?
3.  What findings would be expected at the time of heart catheterization?
4.  What therapy, other than digitalis, diuretics and vasodilators, is indicated?

ANSWERS

1. A diagnosis of left ventricular aneurysm is strongly suggested by the history of a large infarction, repeated episodes of congestive heart failure, and an ECG with persistent ST elevation.
2. The diagnosis is confirmed by findings of dyskinetic wall motion on 2-dimensional echocardiography or nuclear ventriculography.
3. The left ventricular end-diastolic pressure is elevated and often greater than 20 mm Hg. The ventriculogram will show the anterior dyskinetic segment. Coronary angiography may show single- or multiple-vessel disease.
4. A left ventricular aneurysmectomy should be considered. Indications for surgical removal are left ventricular failure, systemic embolization and refractory ventricular arrhythmia.

PEARLS

1. Left ventricular aneurysms occur in 10-15% of patients after a myocardial infarction; most studies indicate aneurysm to be a late complication (months to years).
2. Aneurysms occur approximately 4 times more frequently in the apex and anterior wall than in the inferoposterior wall. Inferior wall aneurysms can cause mitral regurgitation.

PITFALLS

1. A true aneurysm is a well-defined, thin-walled, fibrotic segment of the ventricle protruding beyond the remainder of the cardiac surface. In contradistinction, false aneurysms result from rupture of the myocardial wall, with containment by organized thrombus and pericardium. If a false aneurysm is present, surgical resection should be performed even in the absence of symptoms and complications, because rupture is likely to occur. True aneurysms rarely rupture.
2. A localized well-healed aneurysm in an asymptomatic patient with single-vessel coronary artery disease (CAD) requires no other treatment than that which usually accompanies CAD.
3. Simple left ventricular aneurysmectomy has demonstrated only limited success in patients with aneurysms and malignant ventricular arrhythmia. The addition of endocardial resection and/or ablative

surgery guided by intraoperative mapping has substantially improved the success of arrhythmia surgery.

## REFERENCES

Bulkley B: Pathophysiology of Coronary Heart Disease. Monograph published, Baylor College of Medicine Cardiology Series, 1983.

Cohen M, Packer M, Gorlin R: Indications for left ventricular aneurysmectomy. Circulation 67:717, 1983.

Faxon DP, Ryan TJ, Davis KB, et al: Prognostic significance of angiographically documented left ventricular aneurysm from the coronary artery surgery study (CASS). Am J Cardiol 50:157, 1982.

Rowe G: Ventricular aneurysms: Current concepts. Hosp Med 21:21, 1985.

## TABLE OF CONTENTS BY DIAGNOSIS

CASES

# Index